Obesity is a complex medical disease which puts you at risk for numerous other diseases. It has been shown to increase disability, decrease the length of your life, and may prevents you from living up to your highest potential- robbing the world of your unique gifts.

I have created this journal as a sacred space for you to work through your challenges of obesity. You will find over 80 quotes and weight loss tips to prompt you and inspire you to finally lose the weight.

Please check out the other journals in this 'Healthy Inspiration Journal' series and don't forget to leave a review on Amazon so others may find them and gain some benefits.
Your health is your wealth, and I wish you a healthy and happy life.

Diane A. Thompson, MD
www.drdianethompson.com

# *Thriving Despite Obesity Journal*

## From the Healthy Inspiration Journal Series

**Awesome Owner** ...........................................................................

**Date** ...........................................................................

**Healthy Inspiration Journal Series: Thriving Despite Obesity**
**Publisher: PhysicianPreneur**
**New York**

The author made all efforts to ensure accuracy in assigning quotes.

This journal is for educational purposes only and not meant for diagnosis or treatment. Consult with your doctor before embarking on any health or fitness journey.

*If your DNA profile puts you at a higher risk of developing obesity, that doesn't mean it's your fate. You can take control of the environmental side of the equation and reduce your overall lifetime risk by a lot.*

– David Agus

*Getting my lifelong weight struggle under control has come from a process of treating myself as well as I treat others in every way.*

– Oprah Winfrey

_____

_____

_____

_____

_____

_____

_____

_____

_____

_____

_____

_____

_____

_____

_____

_____

_____

_____

_____

_____

_____

_____

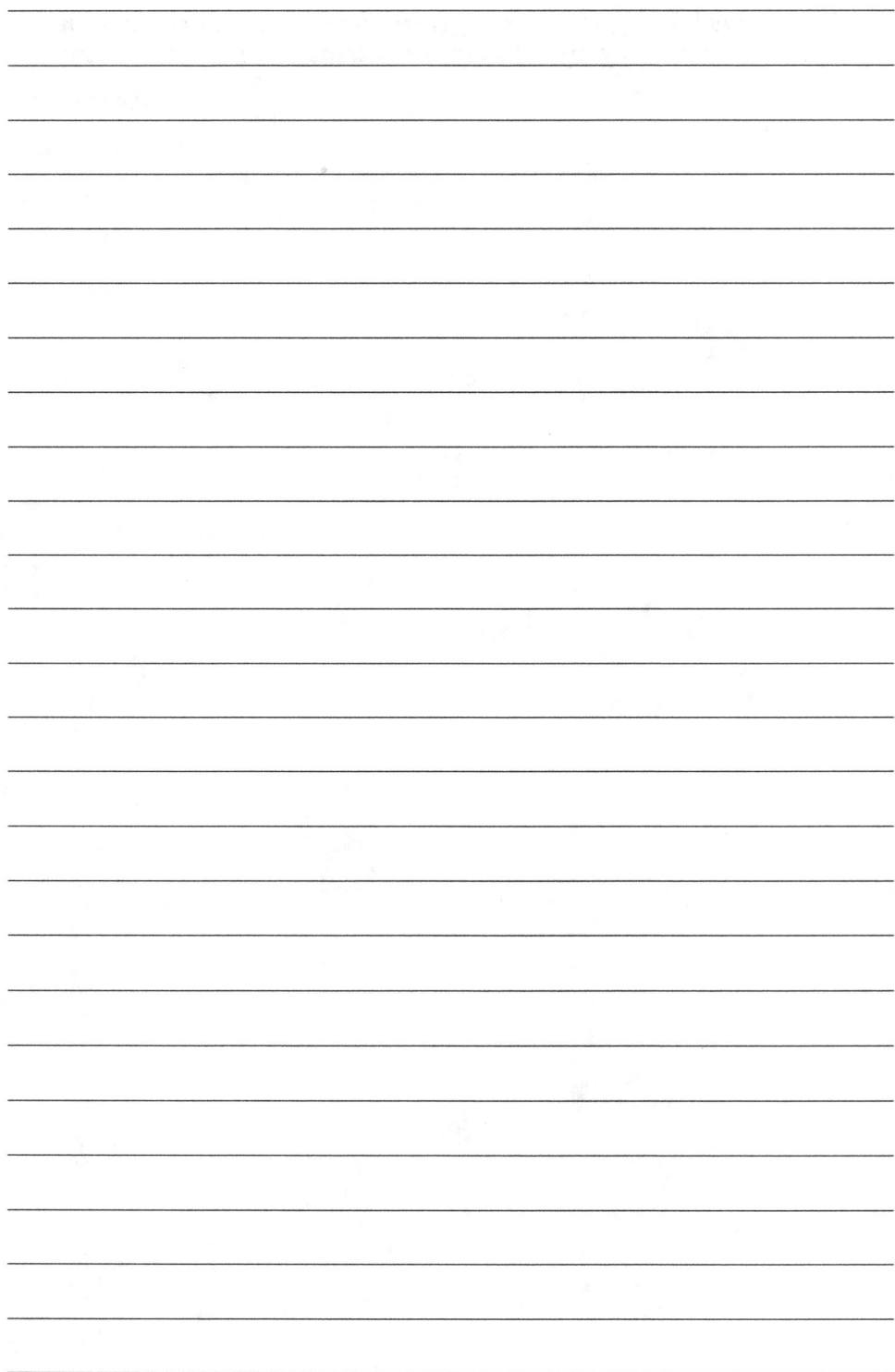

*Tip 1: You are not alone. It is estimated that over 90 million Americans are affected by obesity and it is expected to climb to 120 million in the next 5 years.*

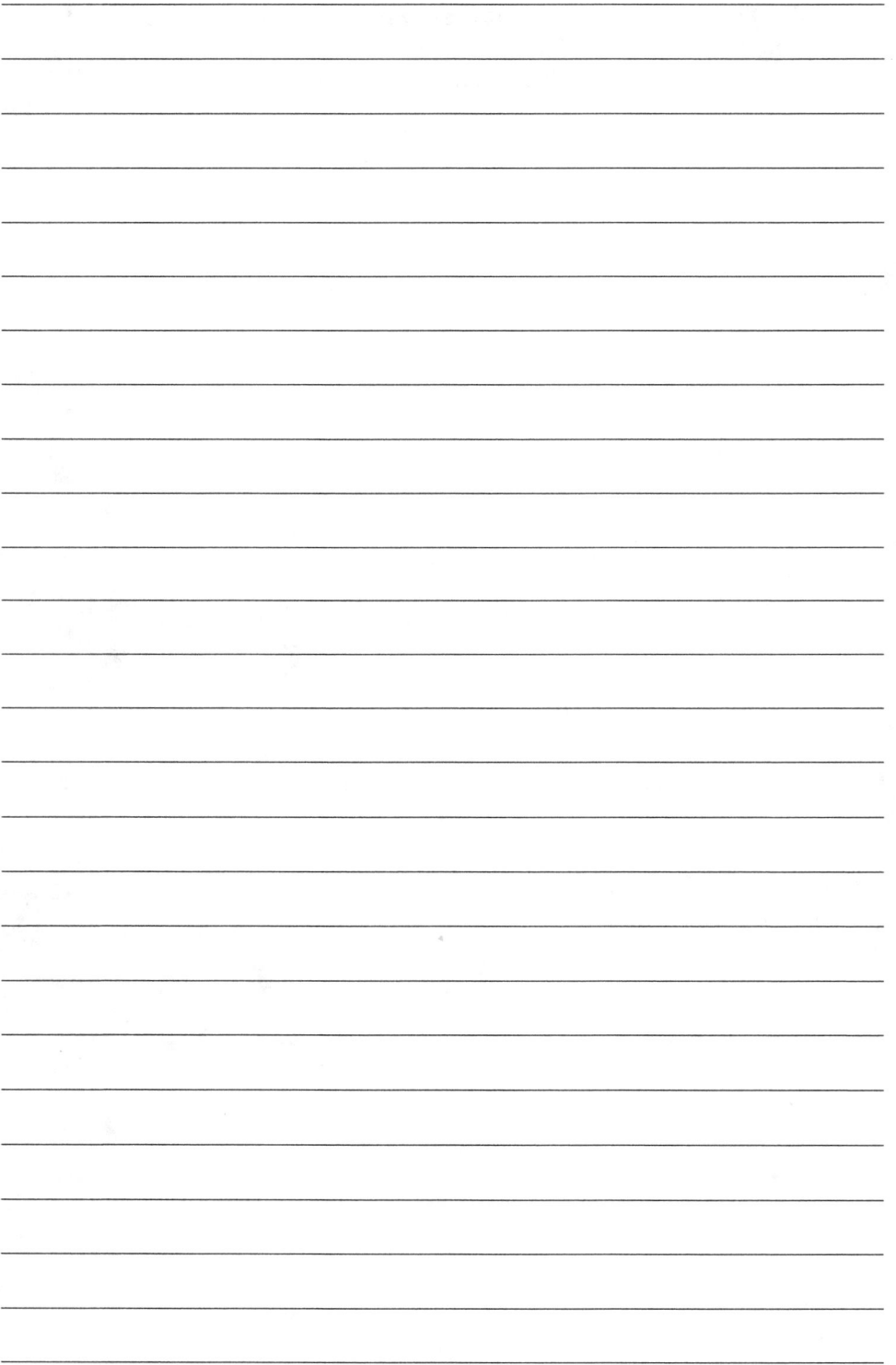

*The key thing is figuring out what your issues are, and it's really never about the food. You have to be real and honest with yourself. I had to stop and look and ask myself, 'Why do I want this? What is the real reason?' At times it was comfort food like chocolate. I love chocolate and I realized it relaxes me, so when you acknowledge what the issue is, you can control it better.*

– Jennifer Hudson

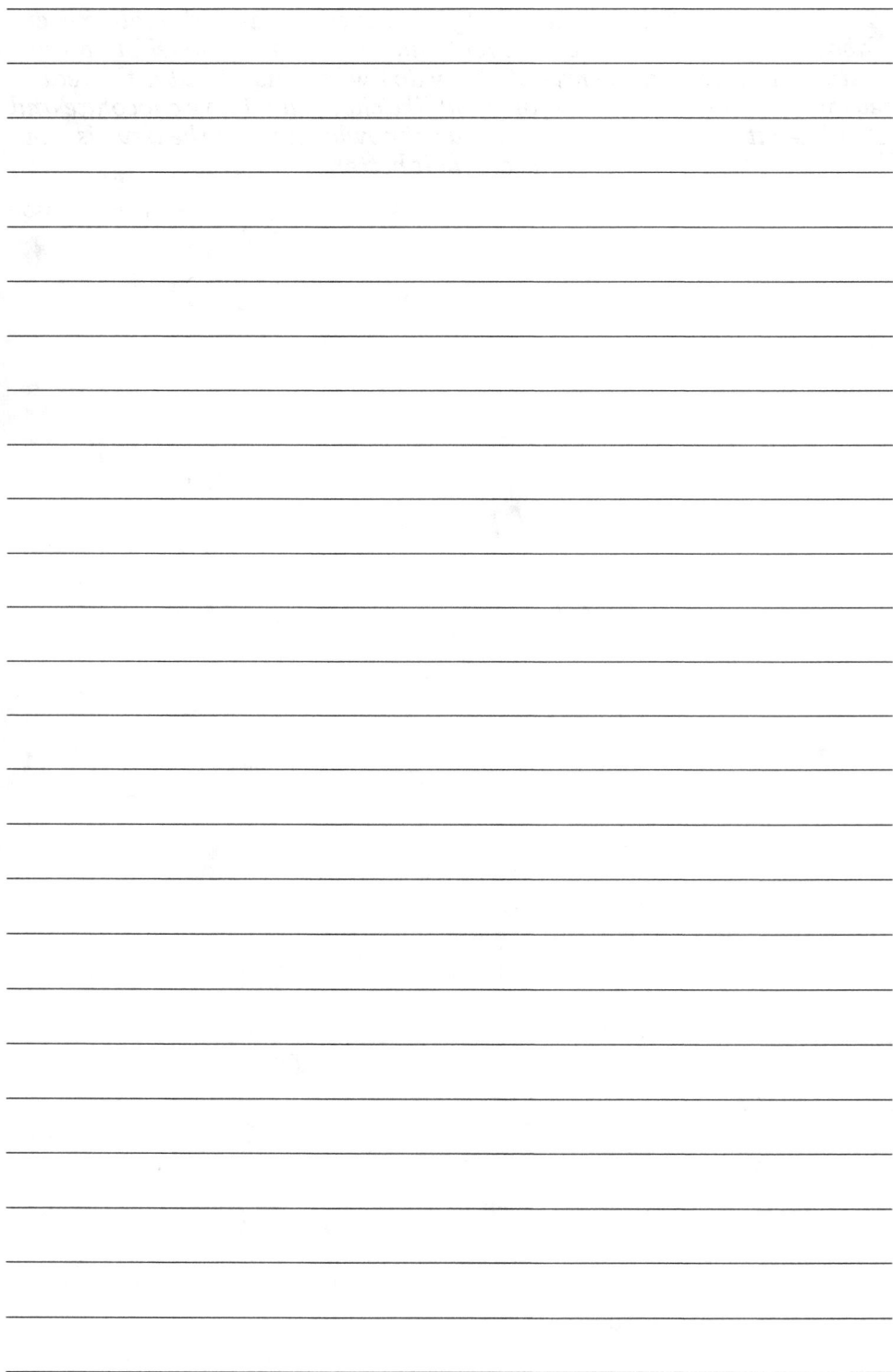

*The way you think, the way you behave, the way you eat,*
*can influence your life by 30 to 50 years.*

— Dr. Deepak Chopra

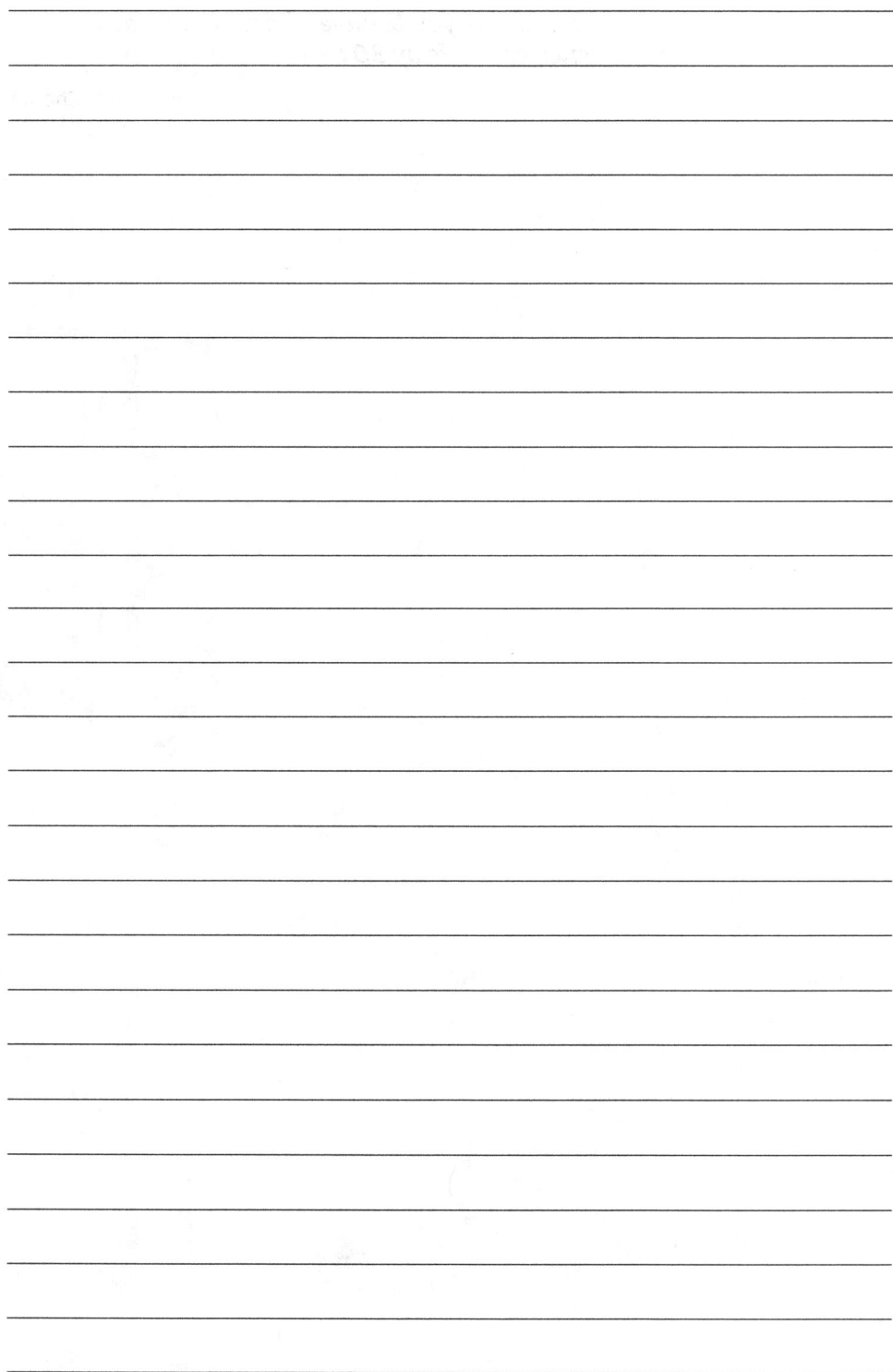

*Remember, we all stumble, every one of us.*
*That's why it's a comfort to go hand in hand.*

– Emily Kimbrough

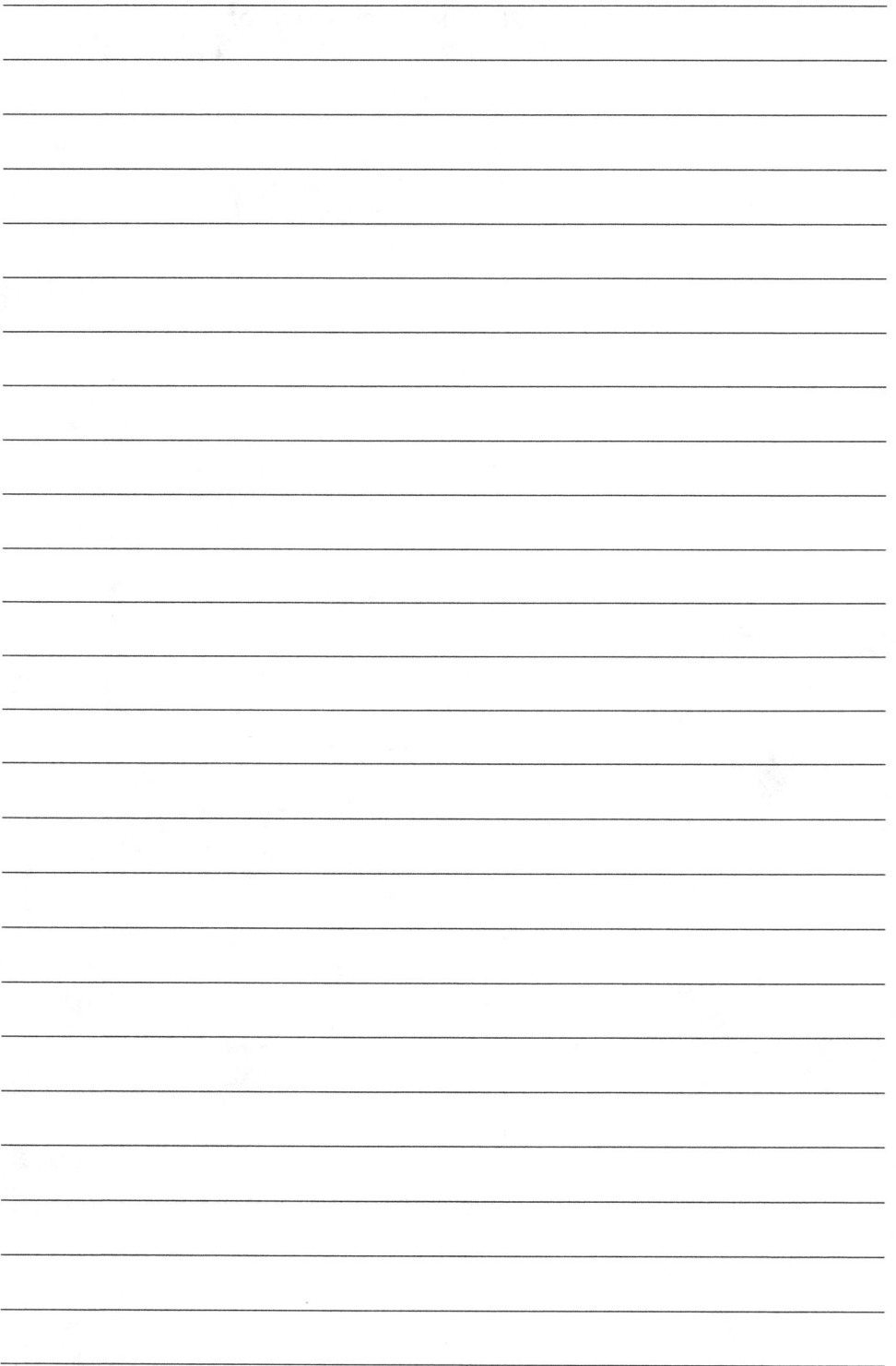

*Tip 2: If you are struggling with obesity, a support group may provide a great way to connect with others who can support and guide you. To find a support group in your area, go to the obesity action coalition.*

http://,www.obesityaction.org/advocacy/support

*Having healthy foods in your home will increase the likelihood of you and your family eating healthily.*

– Diane A. Thompson, MD

_____

_____

_____

_____

_____

_____

_____

_____

_____

_____

_____

_____

_____

_____

_____

_____

_____

_____

_____

_____

_____

_____

_____

_____

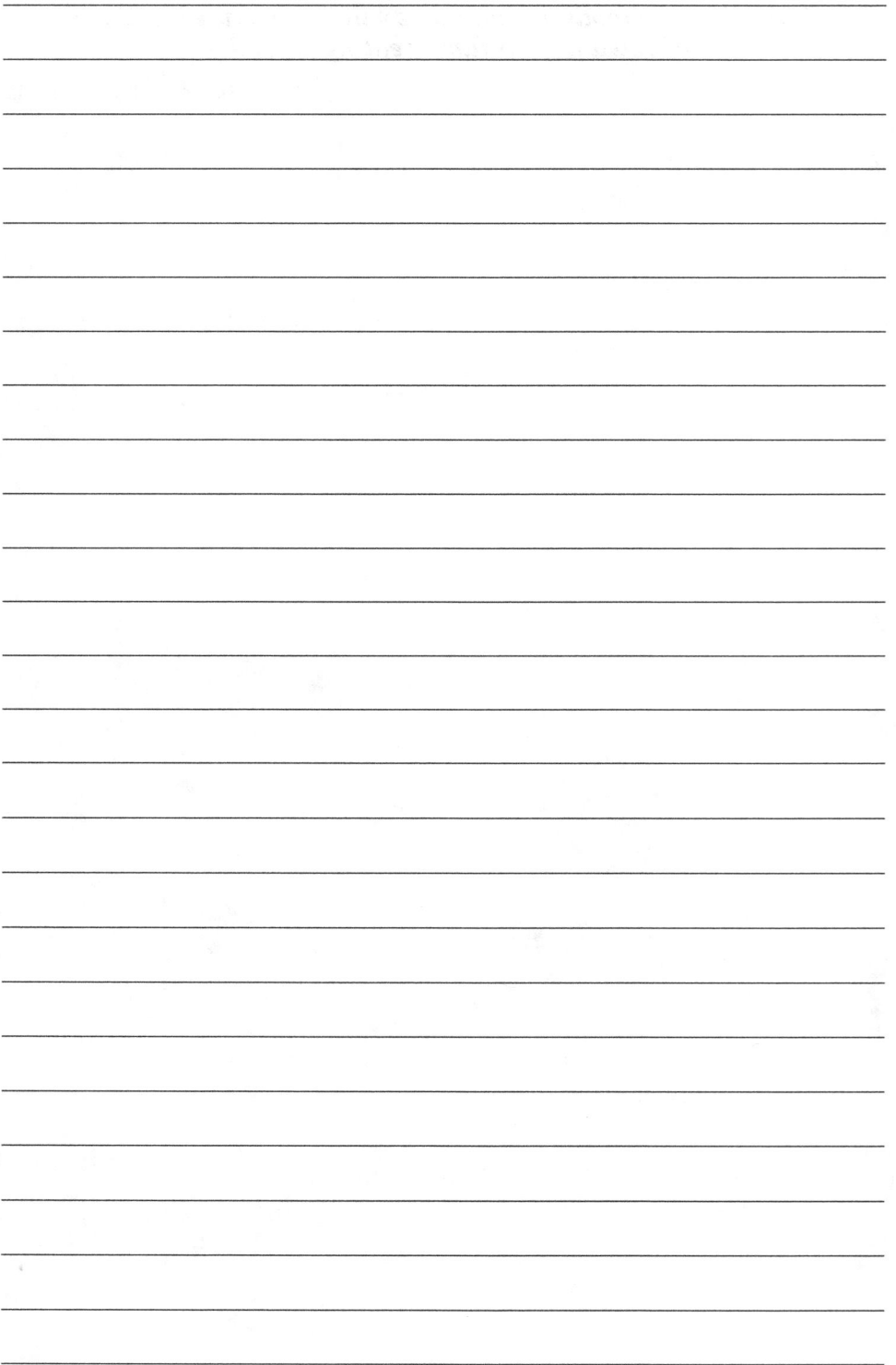

*The rest of the world lives to eat, while I eat to live.*

– Socrates

_____

_____

_____

_____

_____

_____

_____

_____

_____

_____

_____

_____

_____

_____

_____

_____

_____

_____

_____

_____

_____

_____

_____

_____

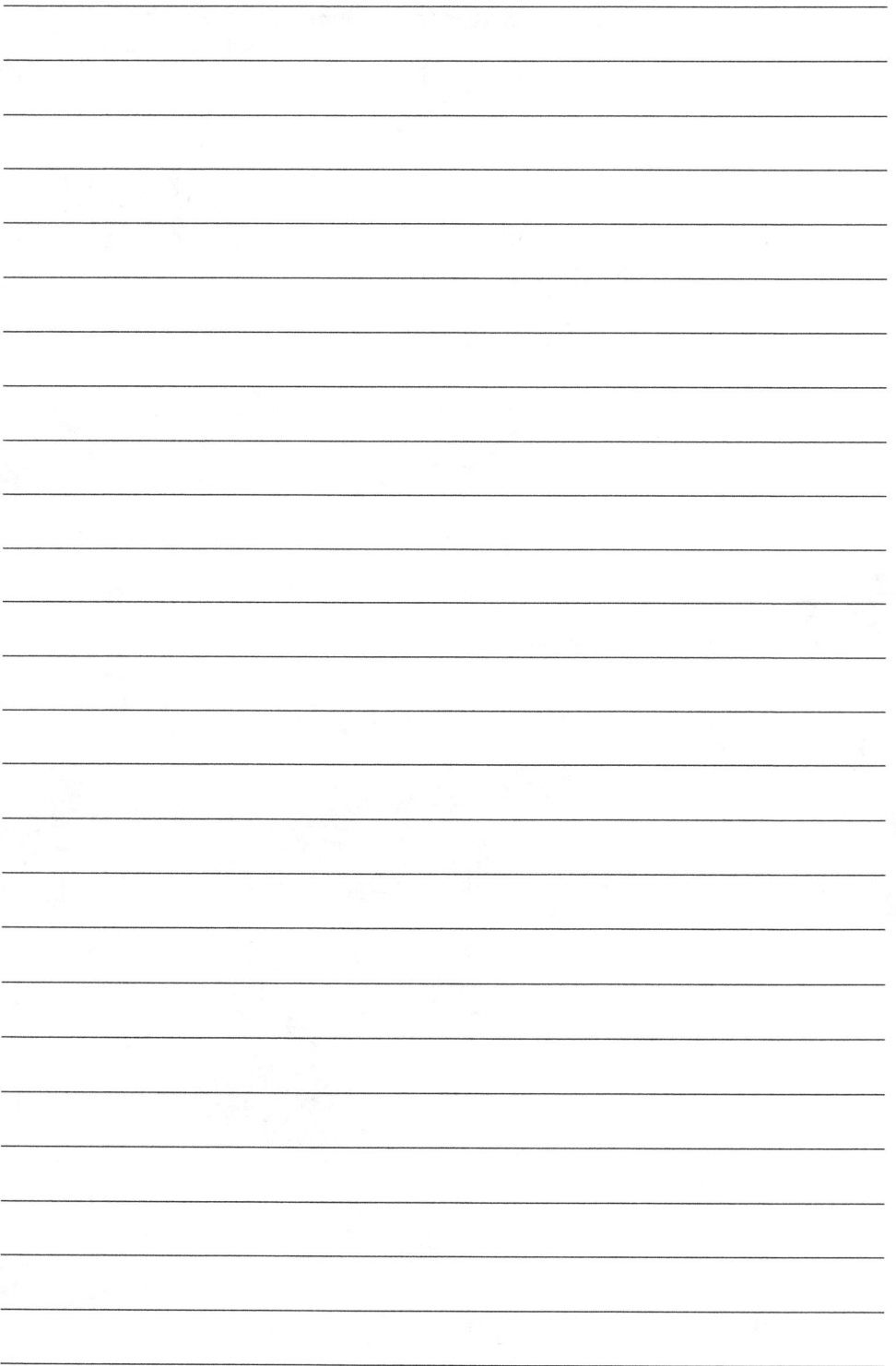

*Tip 3: Obesity is a complex chronic disease that can lead to conditions such as diabetes, high cholesterol, high blood pressure, heart disease, cancer, sleep apnea, poor self-esteem, and disability. Like any other medical condition, it requires self-education and medical attention.*

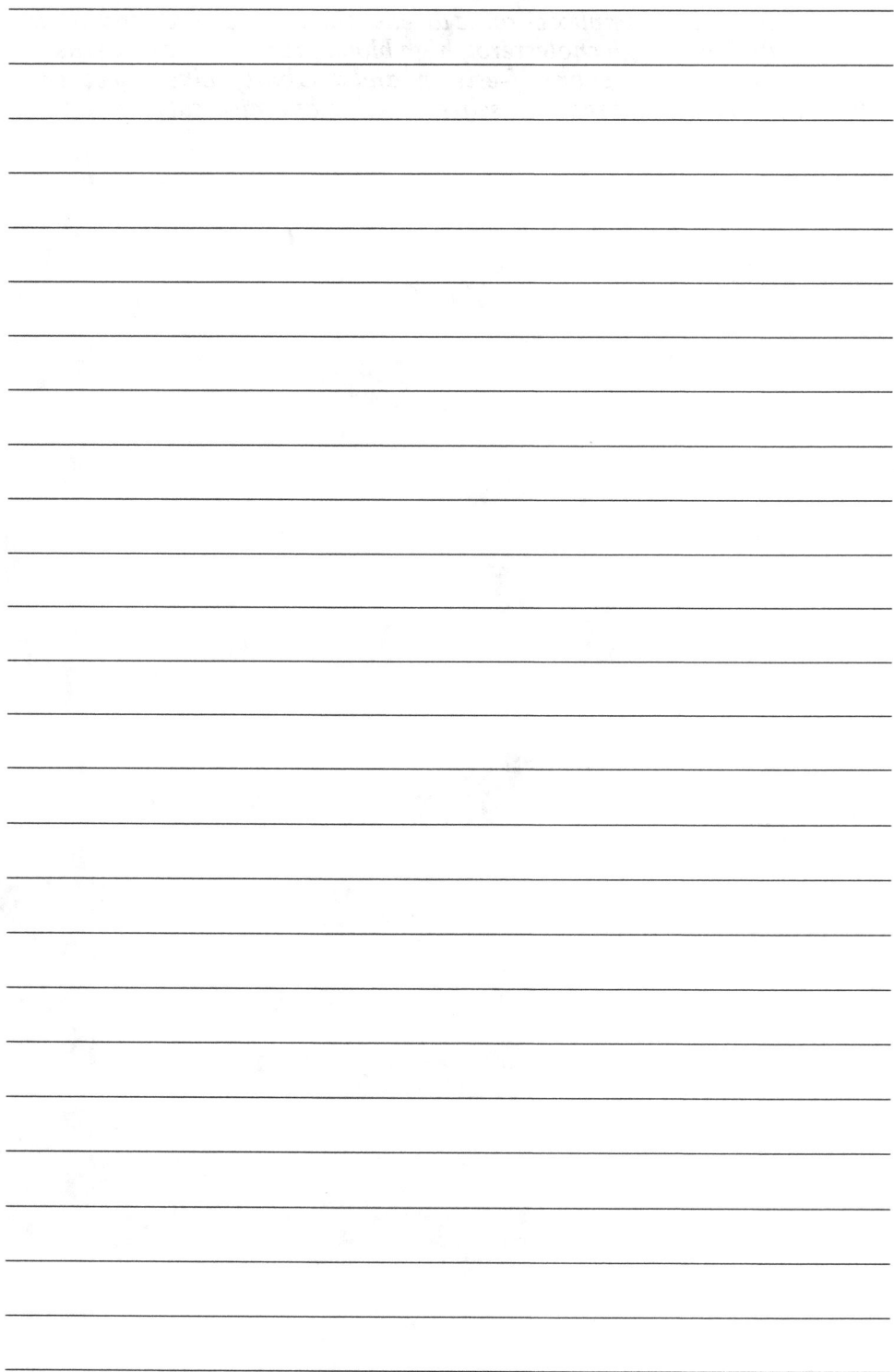

*The physical world, including our bodies, is a response of the observer.*
*We create our bodies as we create the experience of our world.*

– Dr. Deepak Chopra

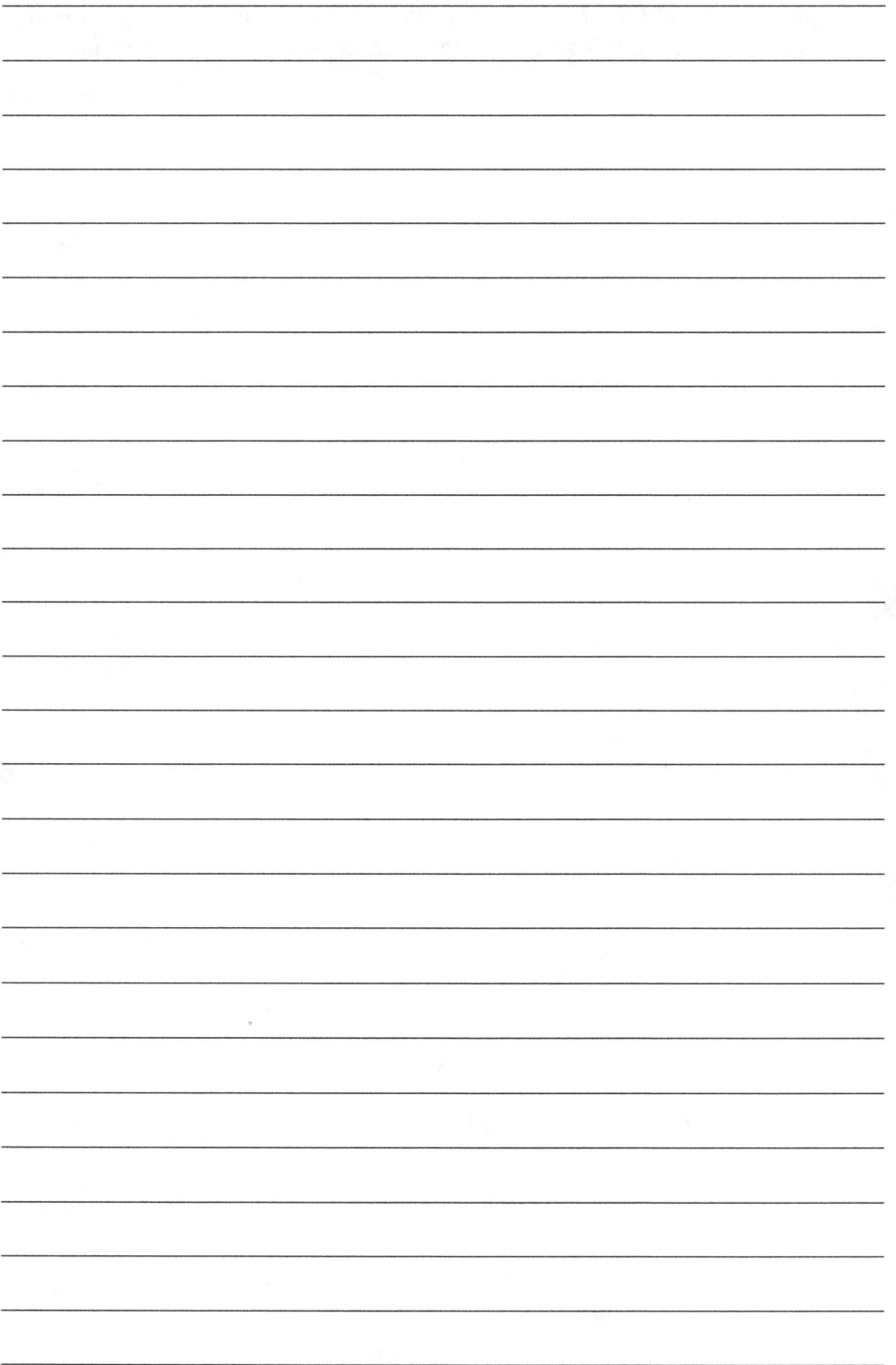

*Eating everything you want is not that much fun. When you live a life with no boundaries, there's less joy. If you can eat anything you want to, what's the fun in eating anything you want to?*

– Tom Hanks

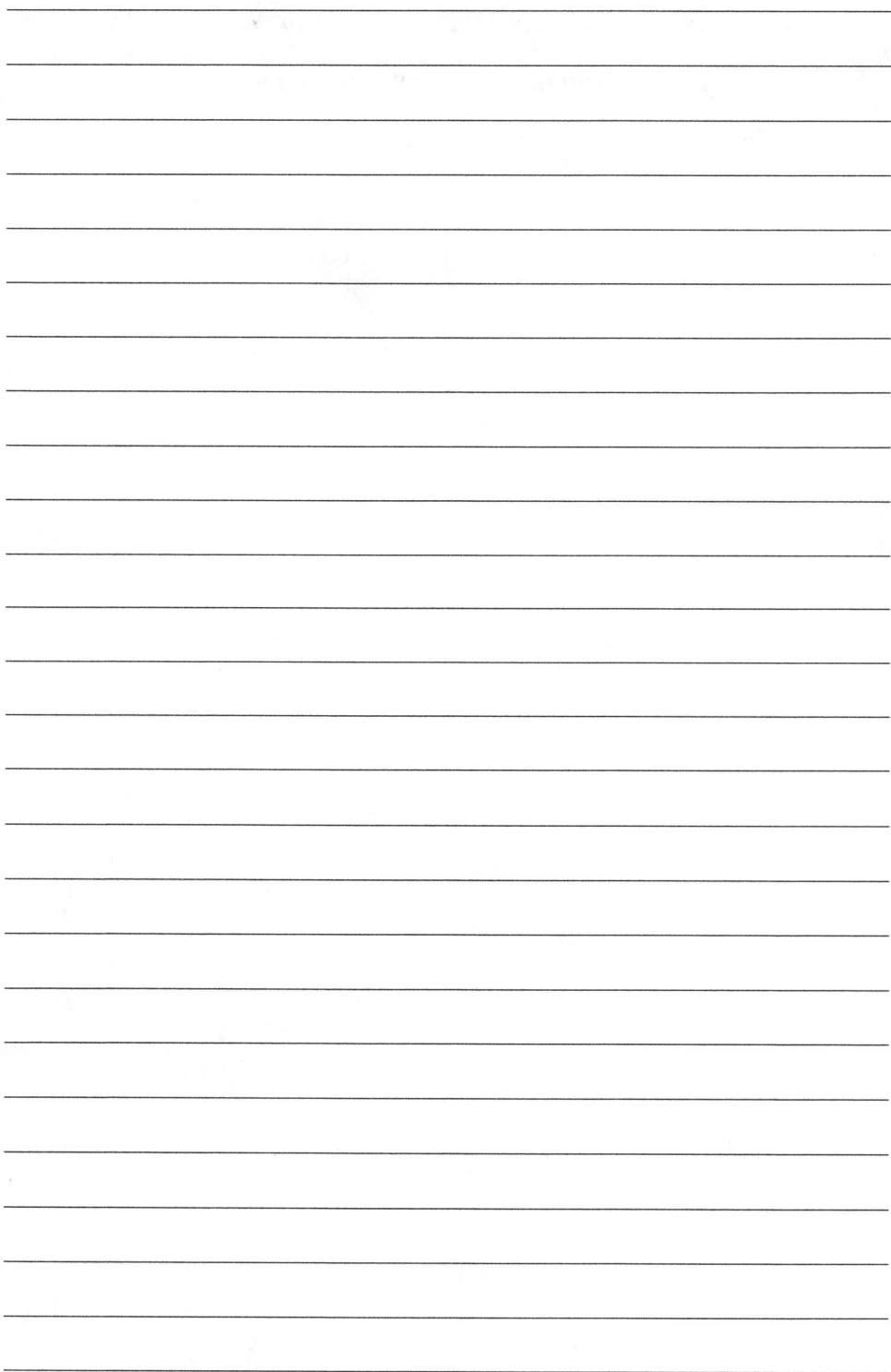

*Tip 4: Drink water, especially before meals.*
*Sometimes thirst may be mistaken for hunger.*

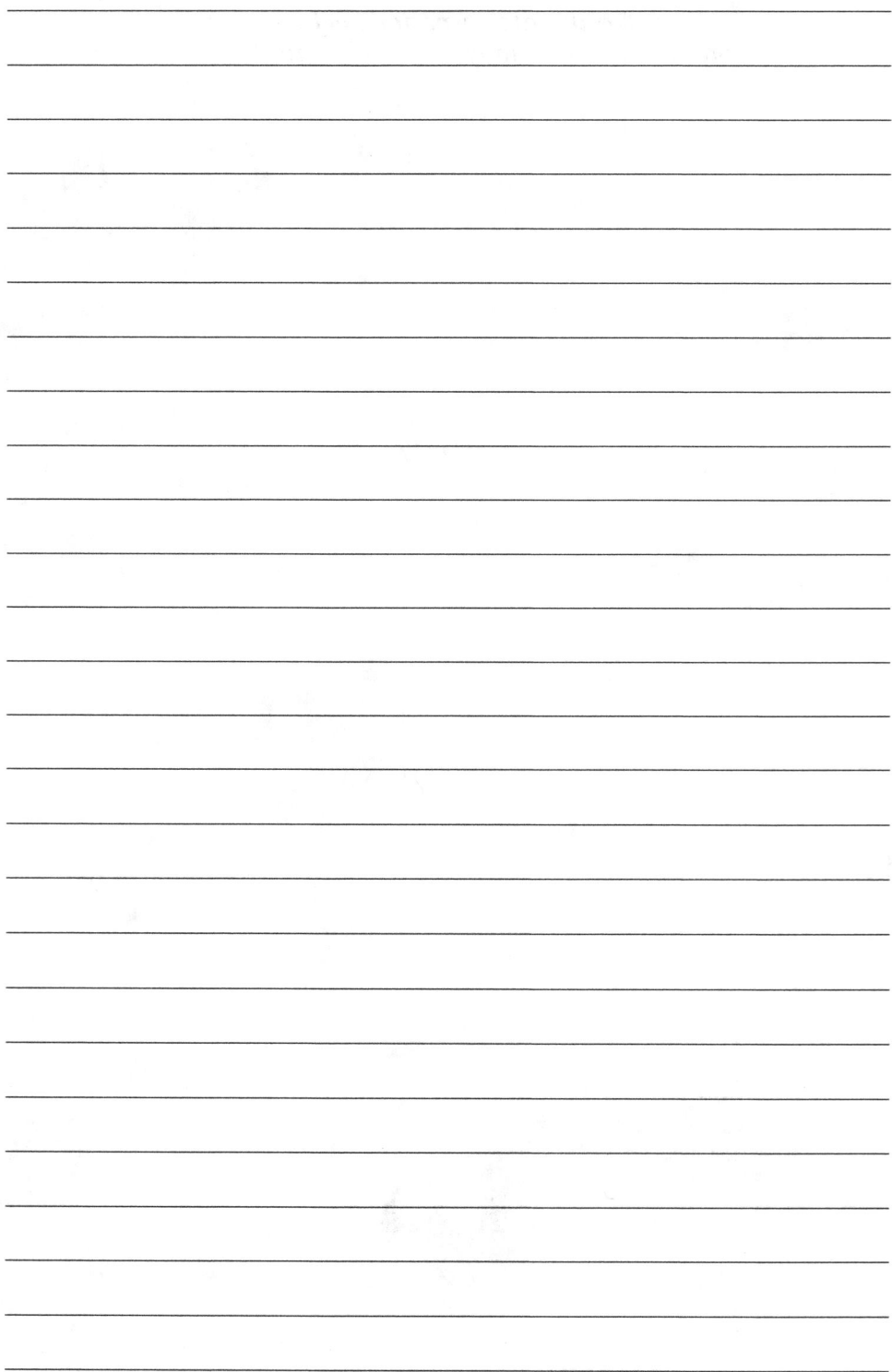

*They will often tell me they can't love themselves because they are so fat, or as one girl put it, 'too round at the edges.' I explain that they are fat because they don't love themselves. When we begin to love and approve of ourselves, it's amazing how weight just disappears from our bodies.*

– Louise Hay

_____

_____

_____

_____

_____

_____

_____

_____

_____

_____

_____

_____

_____

_____

_____

_____

_____

_____

_____

_____

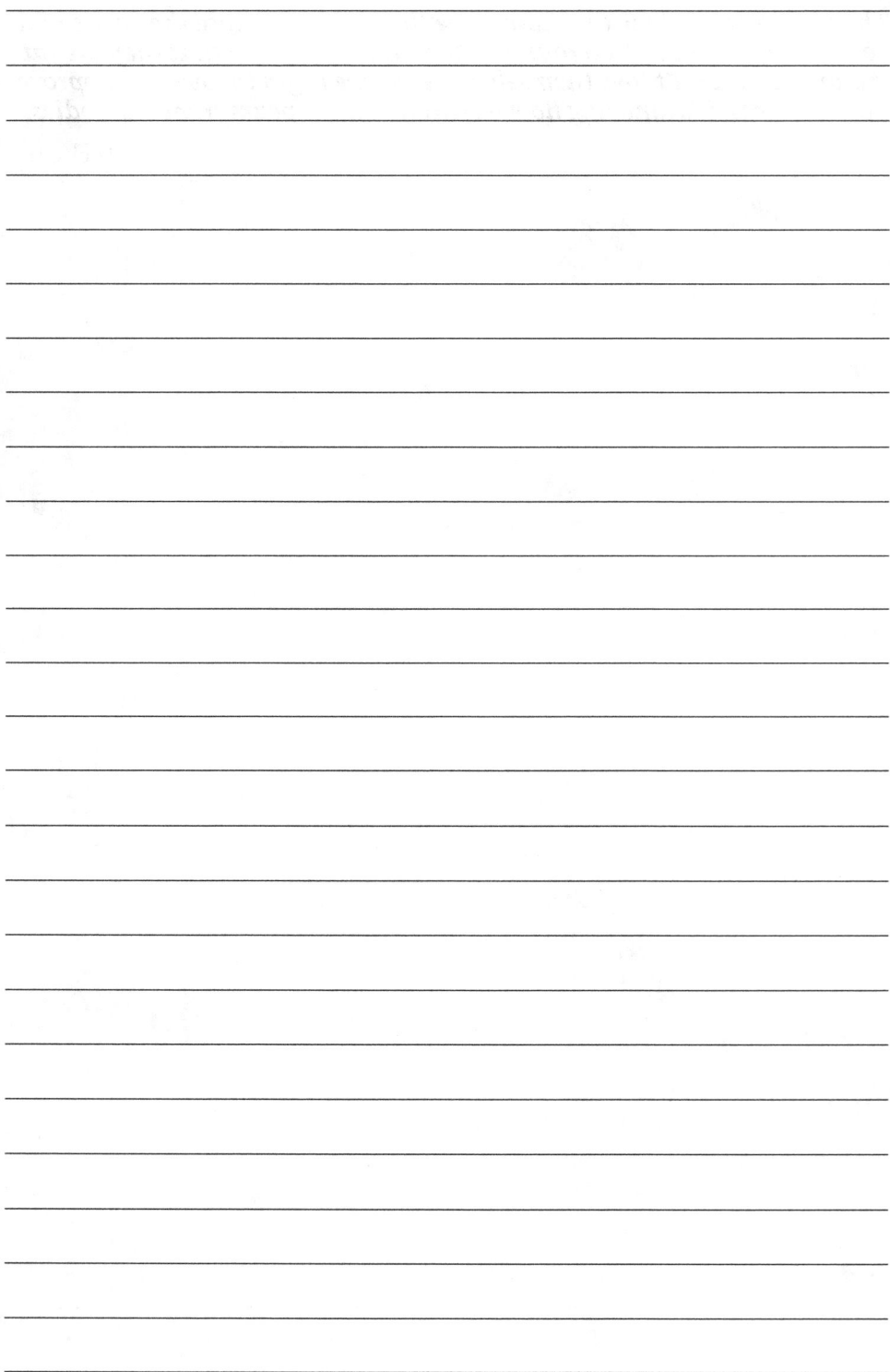

*The one way to get thin is to re-establish a purpose in life.*

– Cyril Connolly

_____

_____

_____

_____

_____

_____

_____

_____

_____

_____

_____

_____

_____

_____

_____

_____

_____

_____

_____

_____

_____

_____

_____

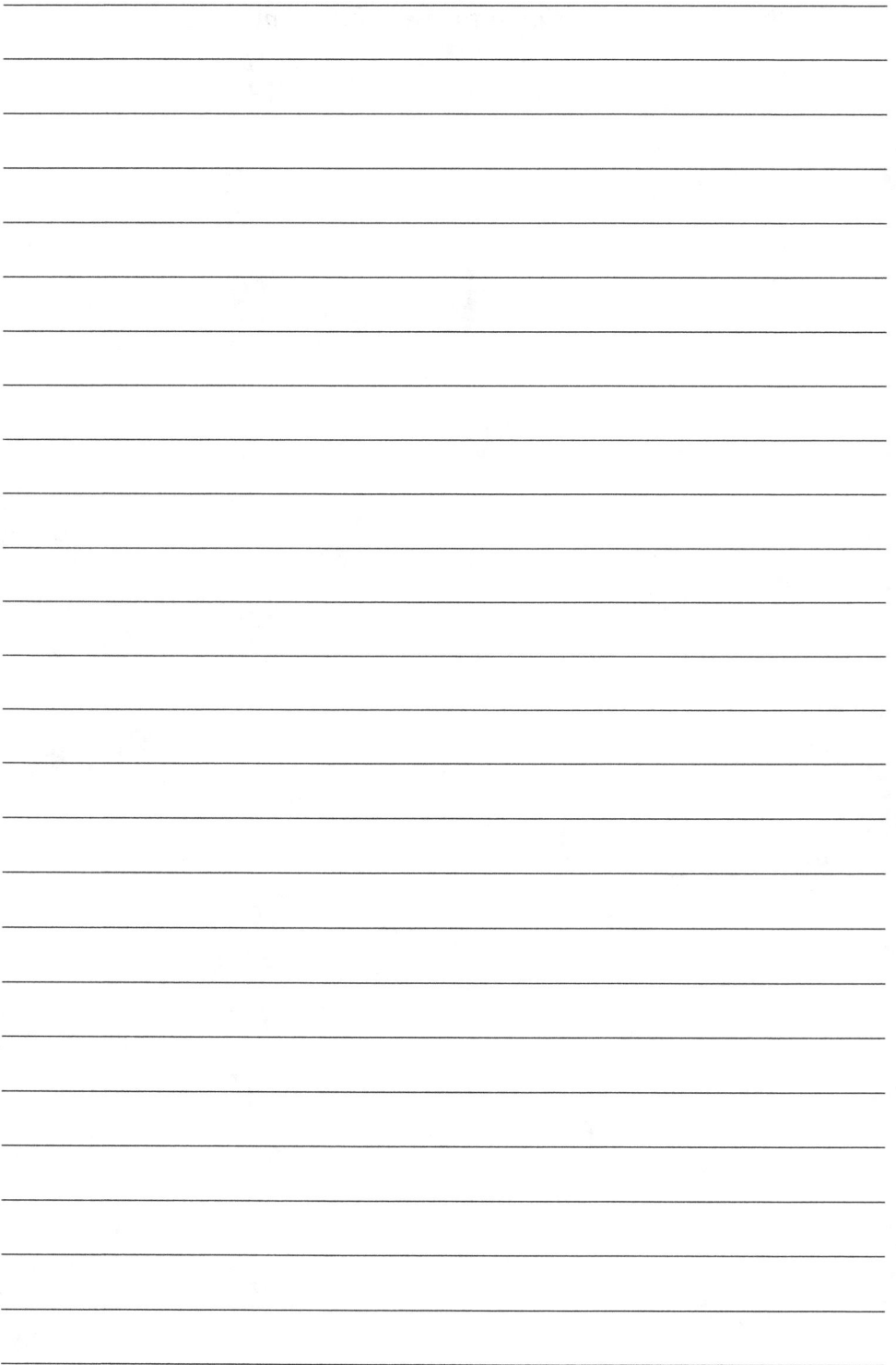

*Tip 5: Add green tea to your regimen. Aside from the antioxidant benefits, green tea is associated with weight loss.*

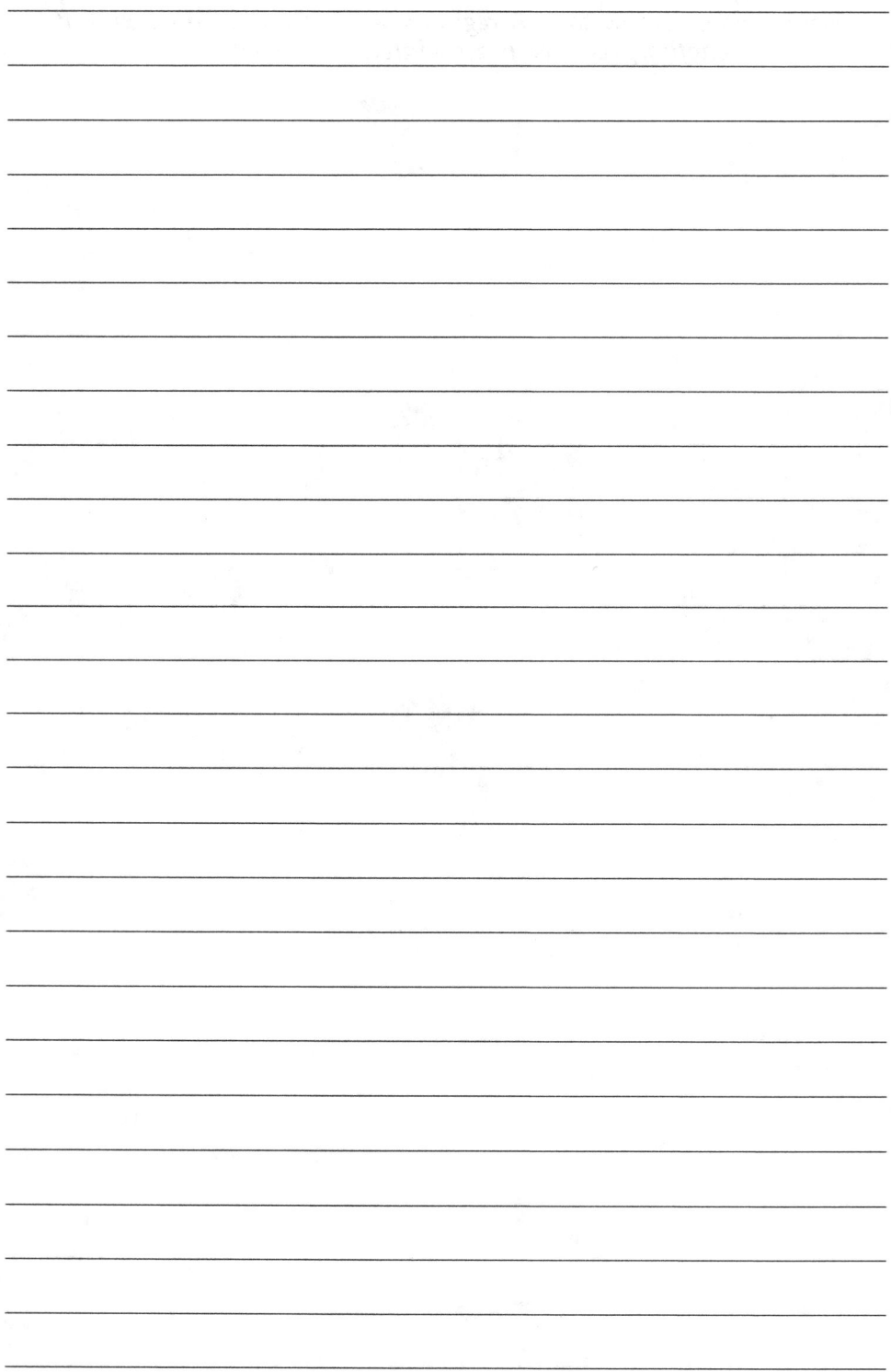

*The doctor of the future will give no medicine but will interest his patients in the care of the human frame, in diet and in the cause and prevention of disease.*

– Thomas Edison

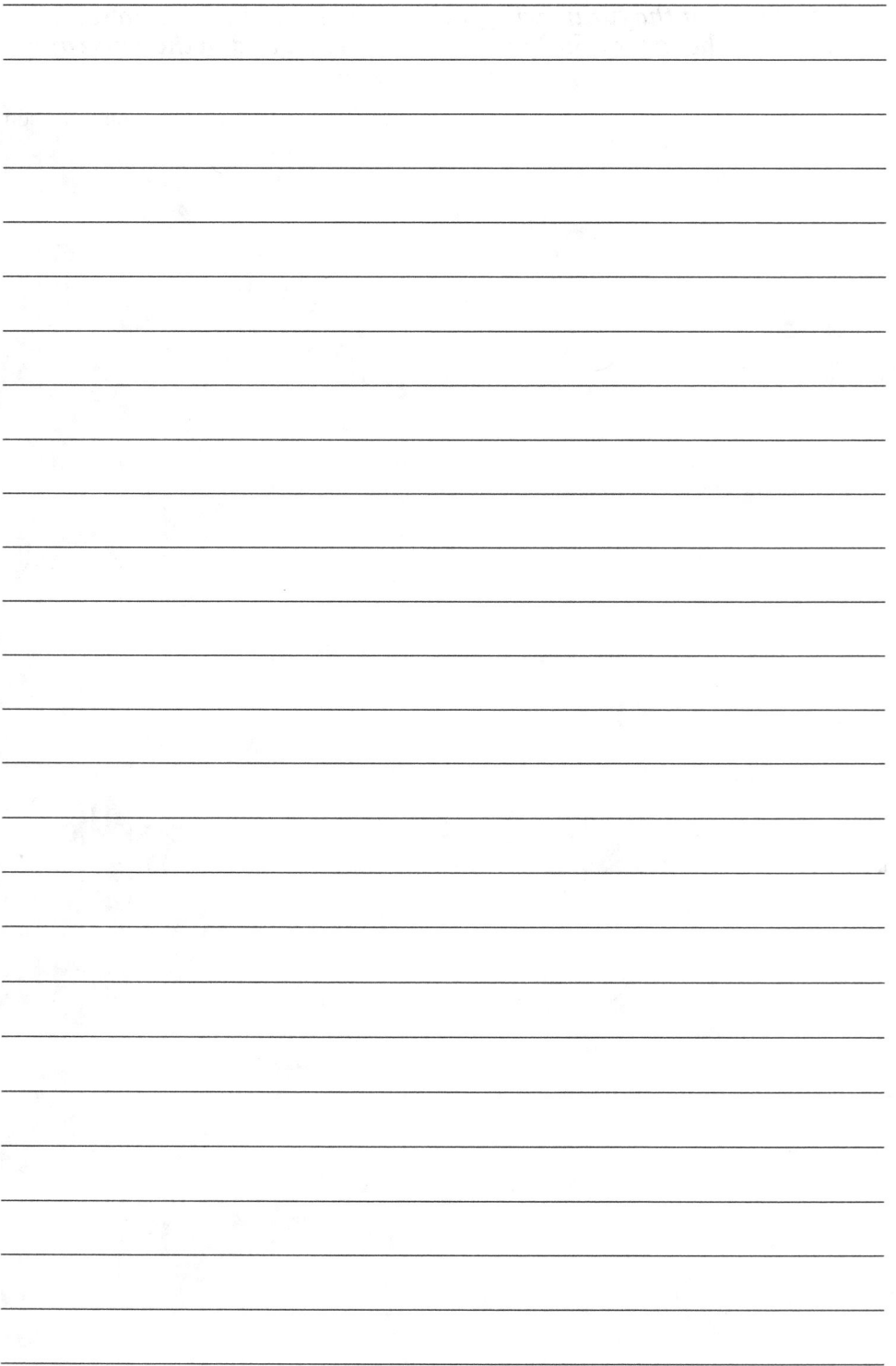

*Take twice as long to eat half as much.*

– Anonymous

_____

_____

_____

_____

_____

_____

_____

_____

_____

_____

_____

_____

_____

_____

_____

_____

_____

_____

_____

_____

_____

_____

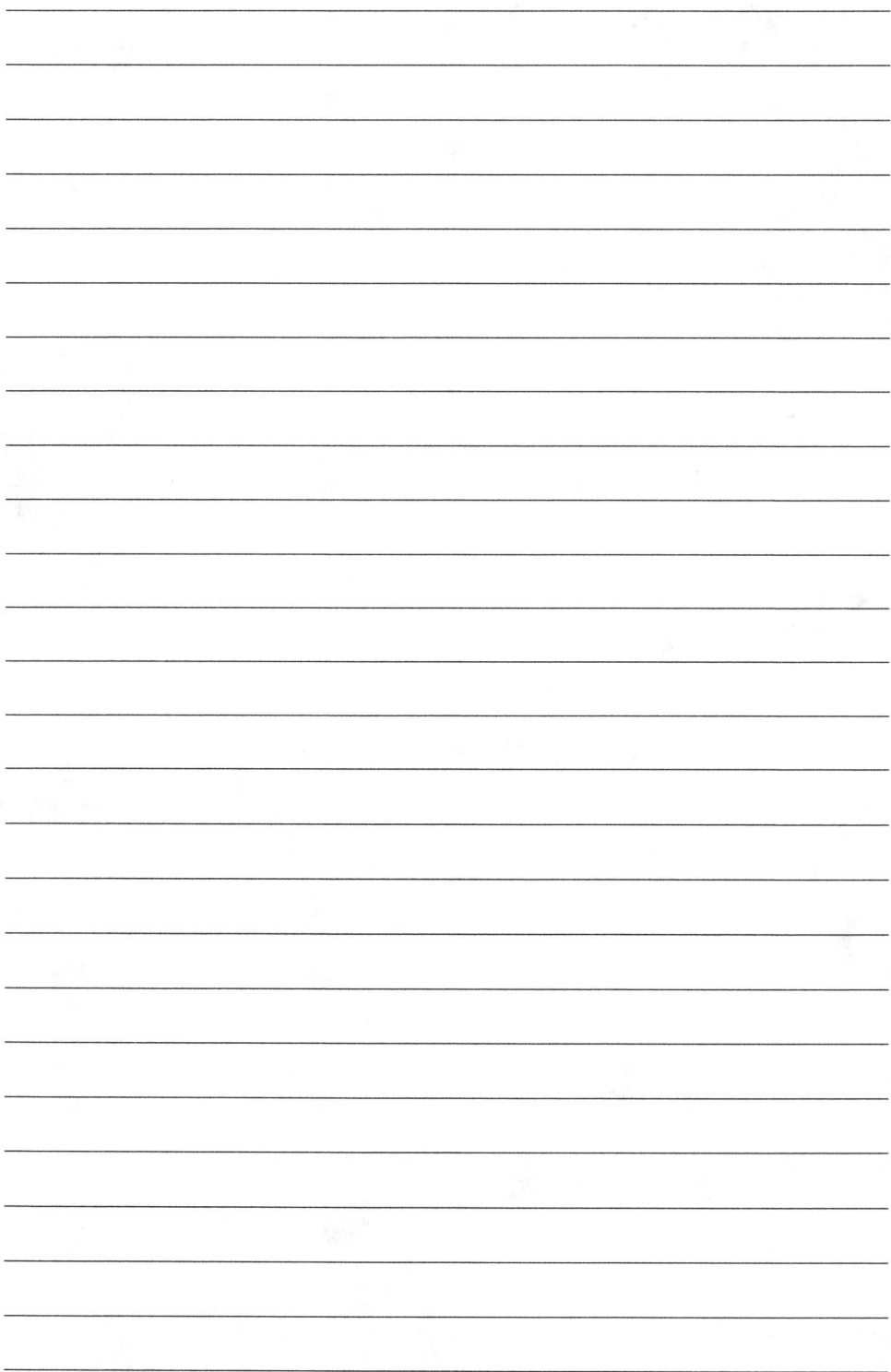

*Tip 6: Decrease your sugar intake.*

_____

_____

_____

_____

_____

_____

_____

_____

_____

_____

_____

_____

_____

_____

_____

_____

_____

_____

_____

_____

_____

_____

*Living a healthy lifestyle will only deprive you of poor health, lethargy, and fat.*

– Jill Johnson

_____

_____

_____

_____

_____

_____

_____

_____

_____

_____

_____

_____

_____

_____

_____

_____

_____

_____

_____

_____

_____

_____

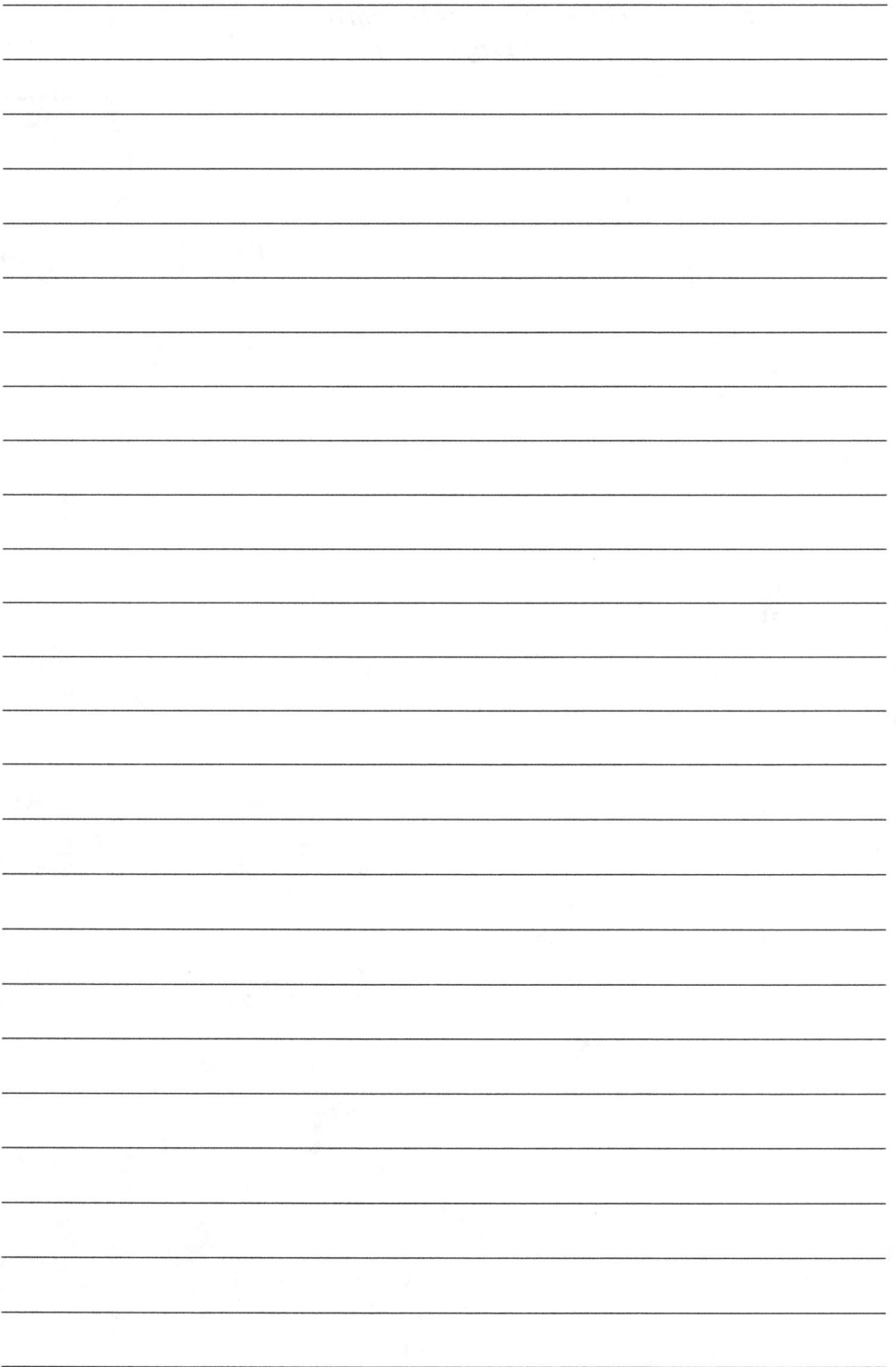

*Take care of your body. It's the only place you have to live.*

– Jim Rohn

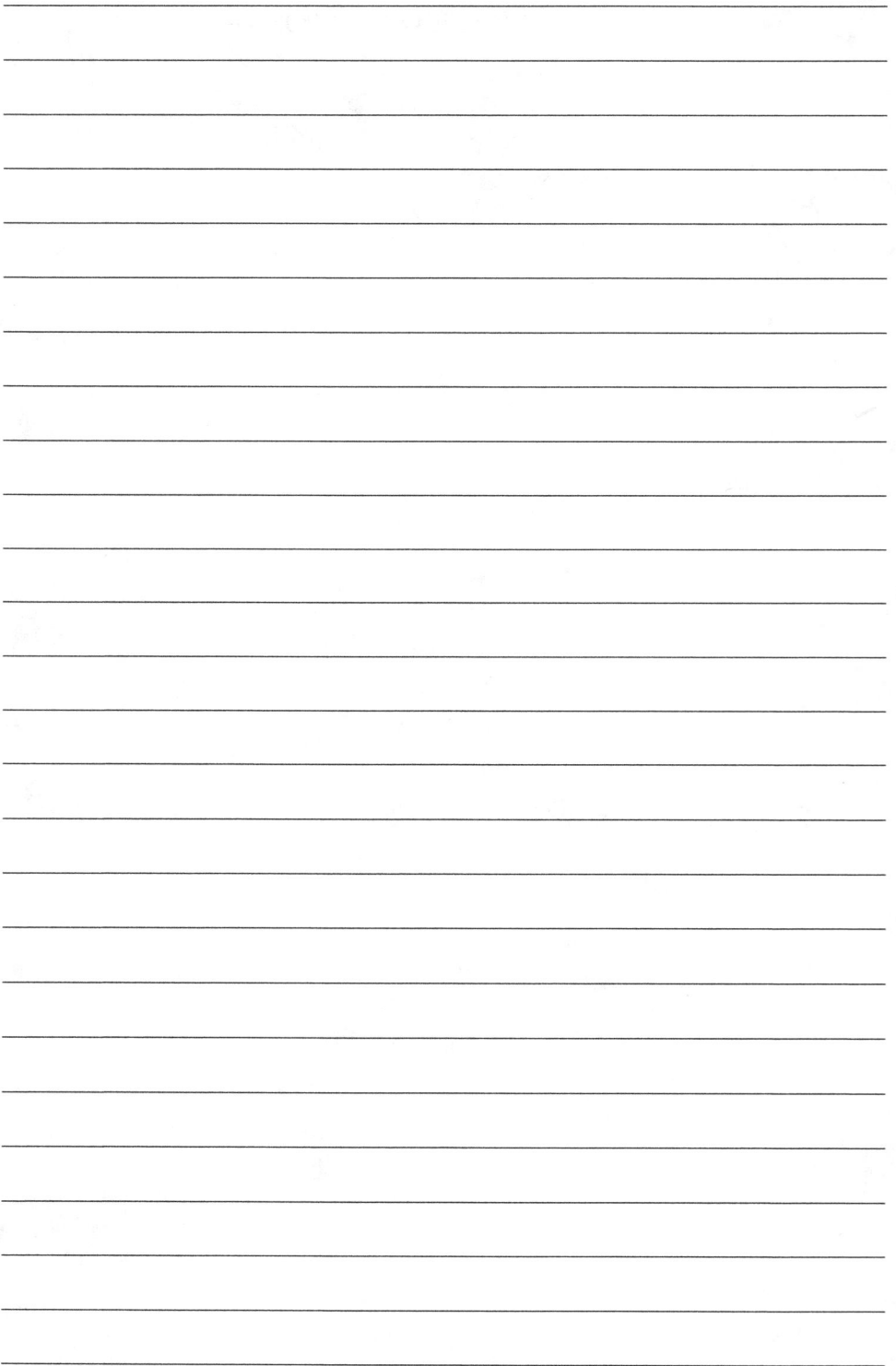

*Tip 7: Add beans to your diet. Not only are beans high in healthy nutrients, they are generally low in calorie, high in fiber, decrease constipation, and helps you feel full so you are less likely to overeat.*

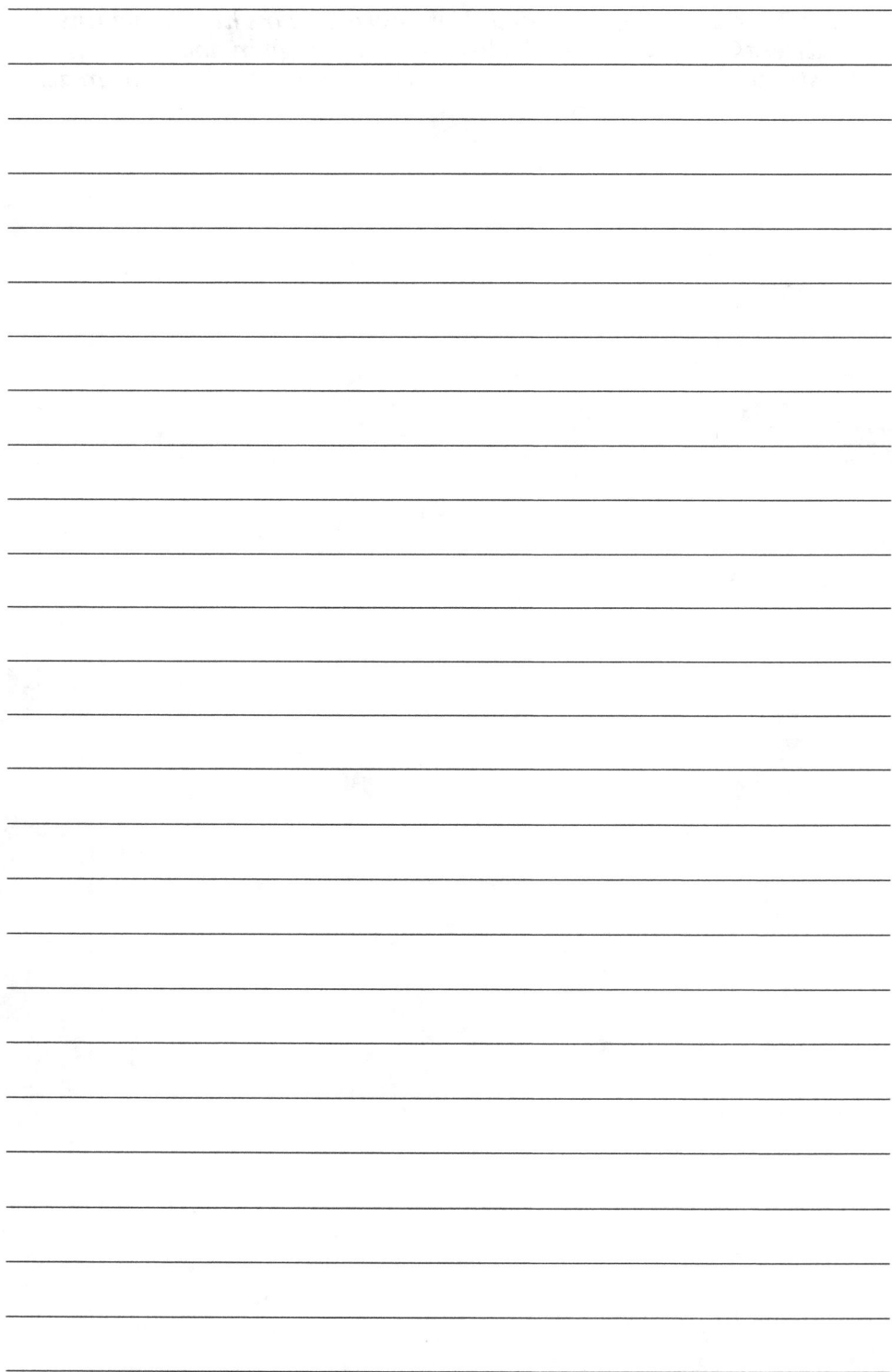

*The big secret in life is that there is no big secret.*
*Whatever your goal, you can get there if you're willing to work.*

– Oprah Winfrey

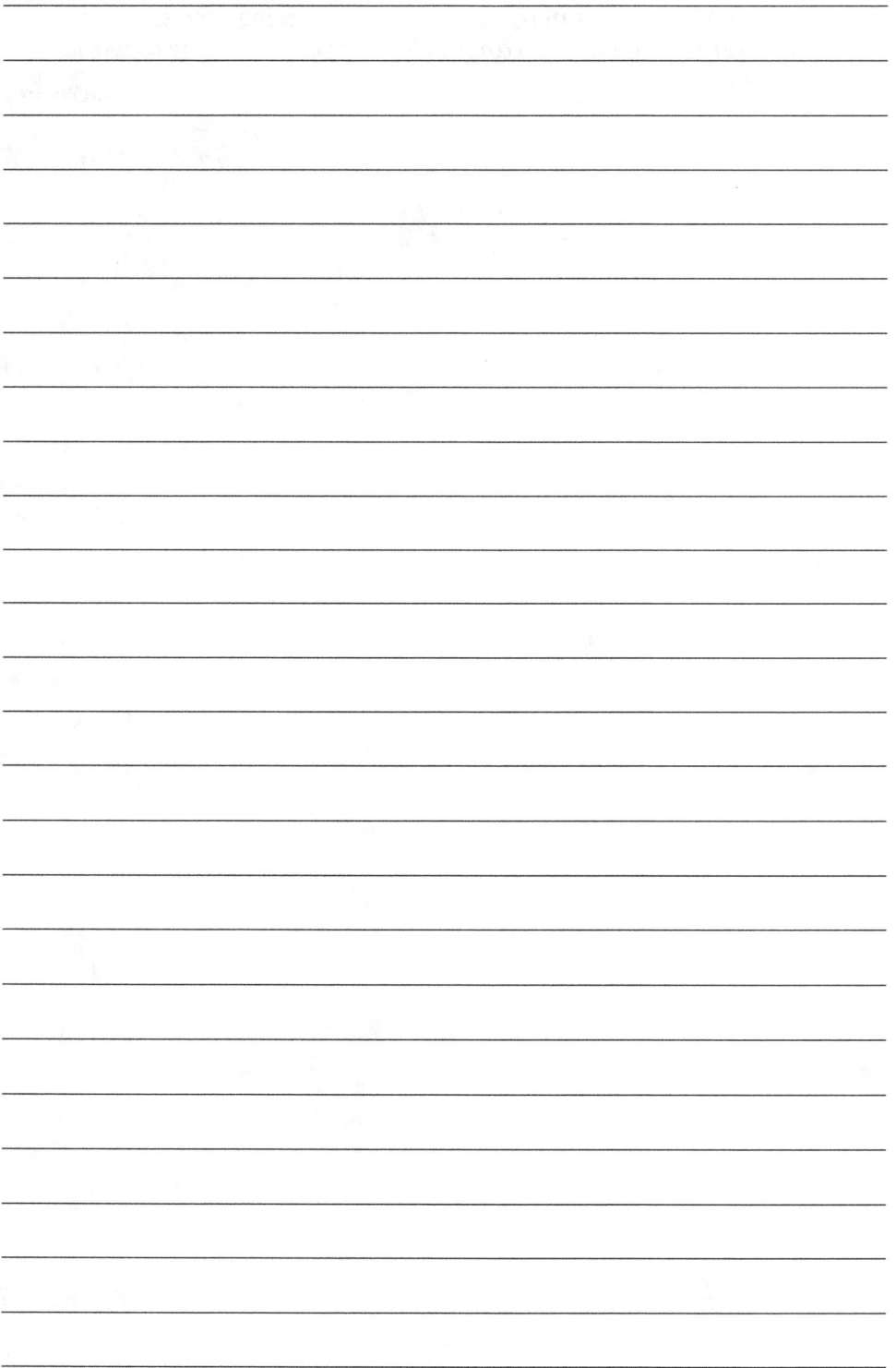

*If hunger is not the problem, then eating is not the solution.*

– Anonymous

_____

_____

_____

_____

_____

_____

_____

_____

_____

_____

_____

_____

_____

_____

_____

_____

_____

_____

_____

_____

_____

_____

_____

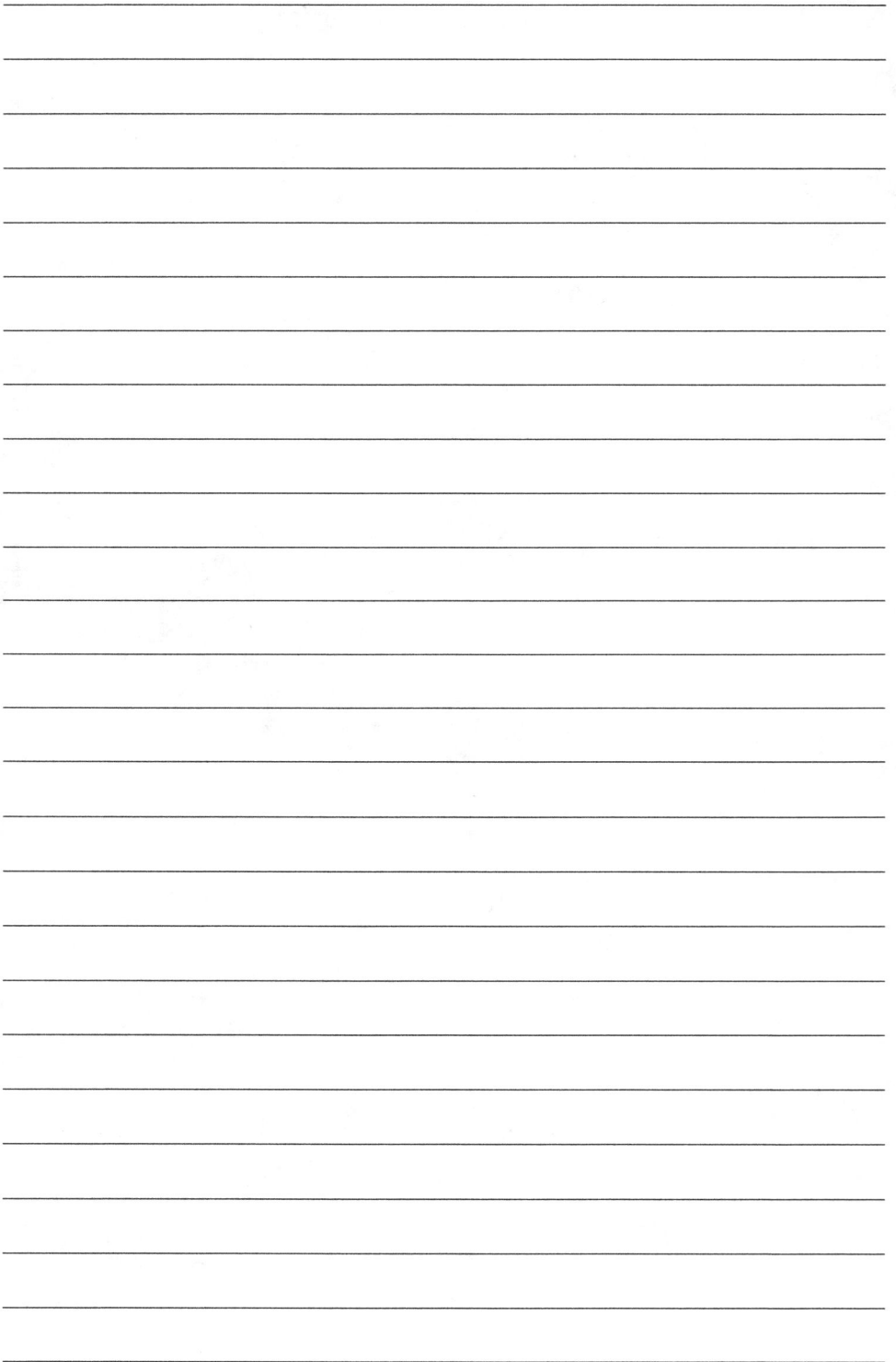

*Tip 8: Eat from smaller plates. Studies show that this helps decrease the amount of food you eat.*

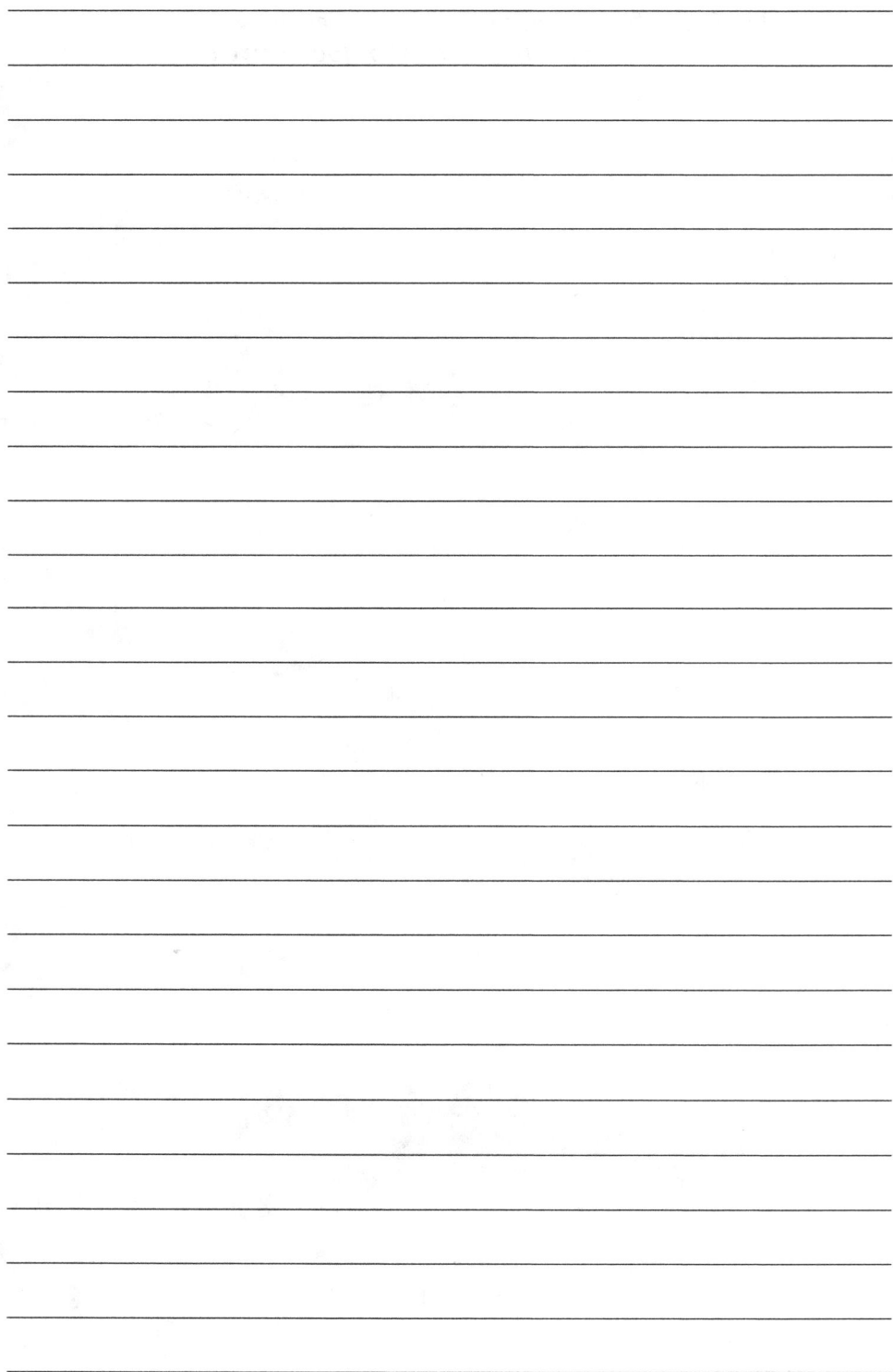

*Every time you are tempted to react in the same old way,*
*ask if you want to be a prisoner of the past or a pioneer of the future.*

– Dr. Deepak Chopra

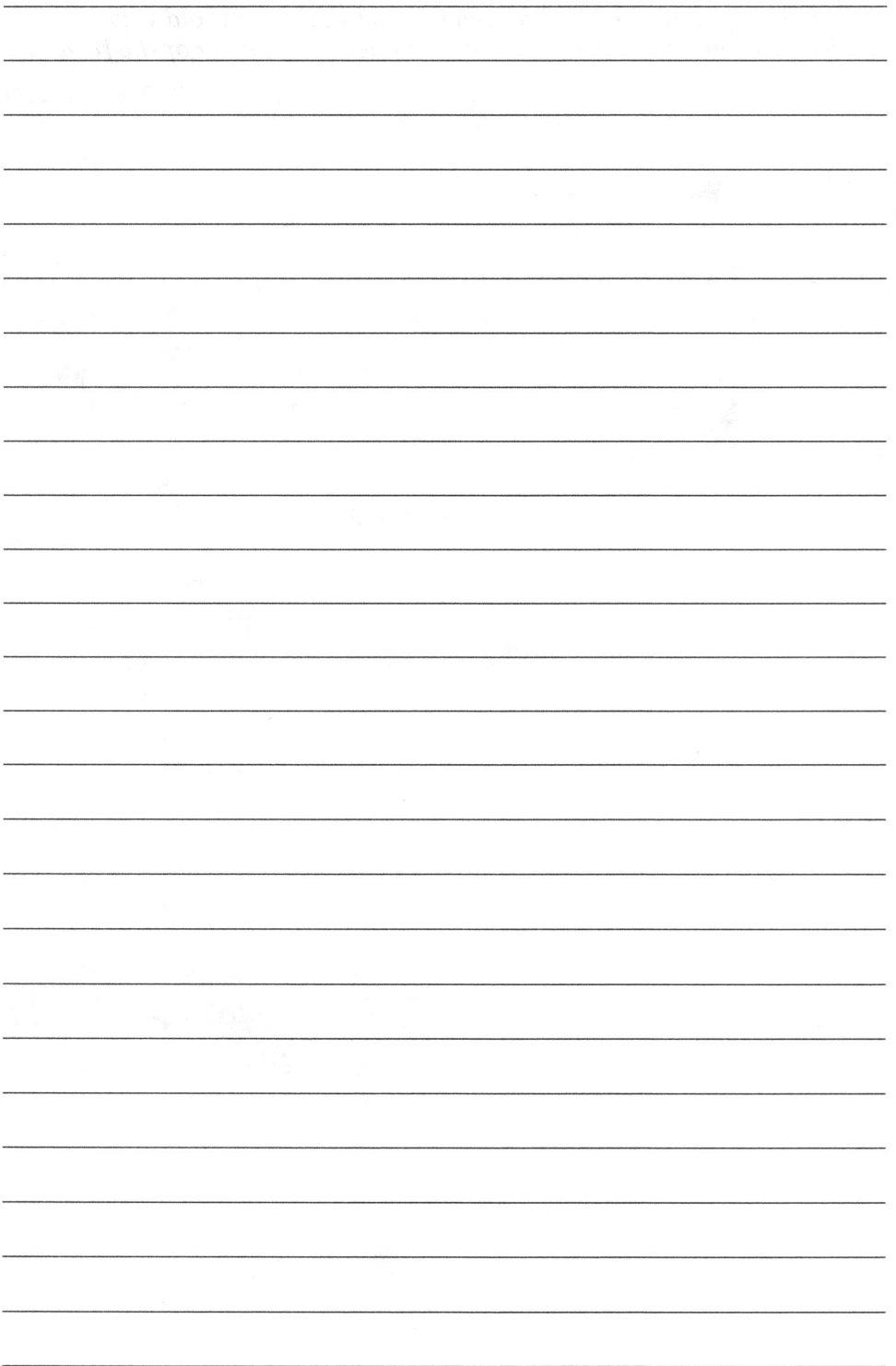

*Reality check: You can never, ever, use weight loss to solve problems that are not related to your weight. At your goal weight or not, you still have to live with yourself and deal with your problems. You will still have the same husband, the same job, the same kids, and the same life. Losing weight is not a cure for life.*

– Dr Phillip McGraw

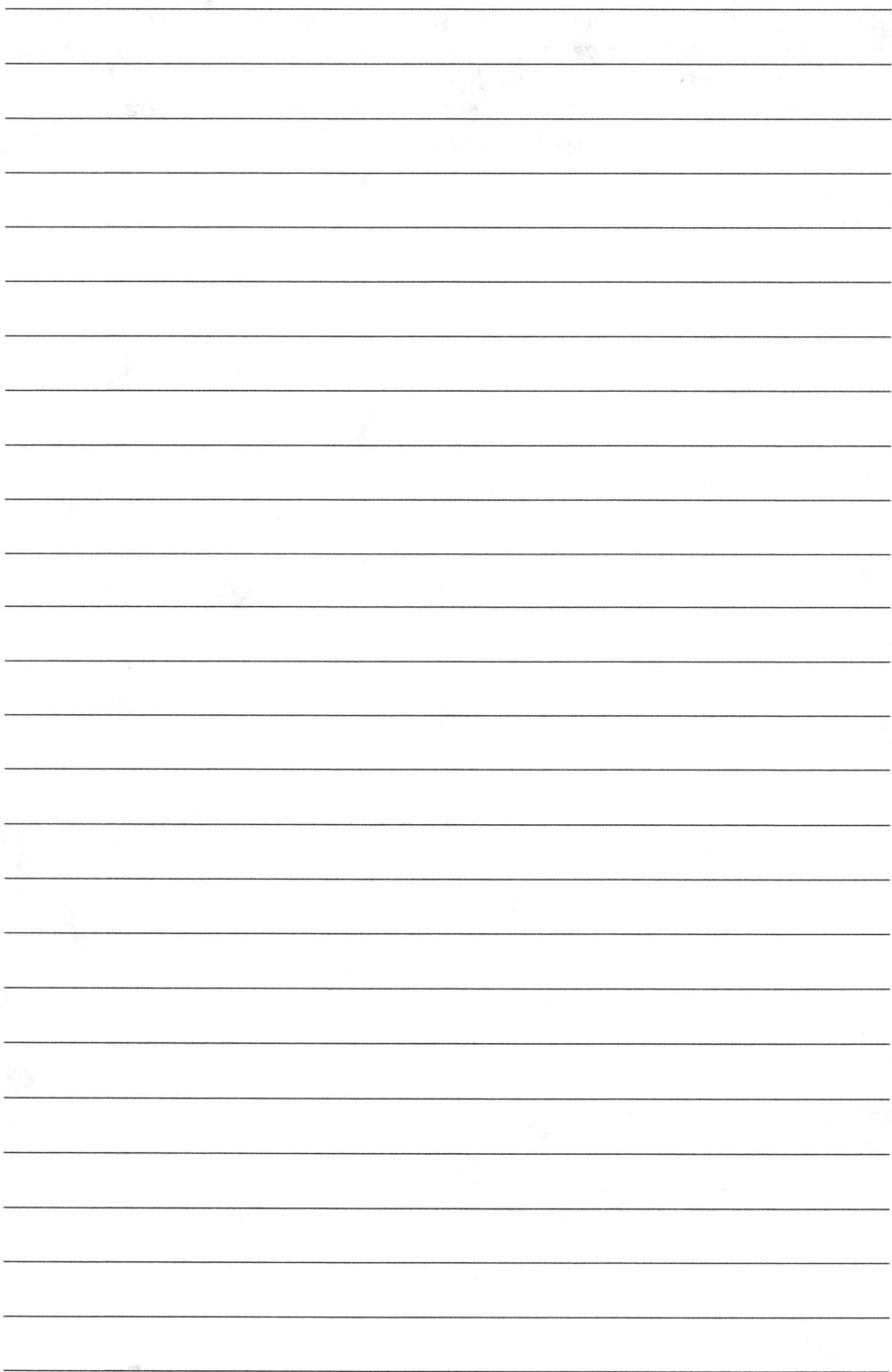

*Tip 9: Keep healthy foods around. You are more likely to eat healthily if healthy food is all you have around you.*

_____

_____

_____

_____

_____

_____

_____

_____

_____

_____

_____

_____

_____

_____

_____

_____

_____

_____

_____

_____

_____

_____

_____

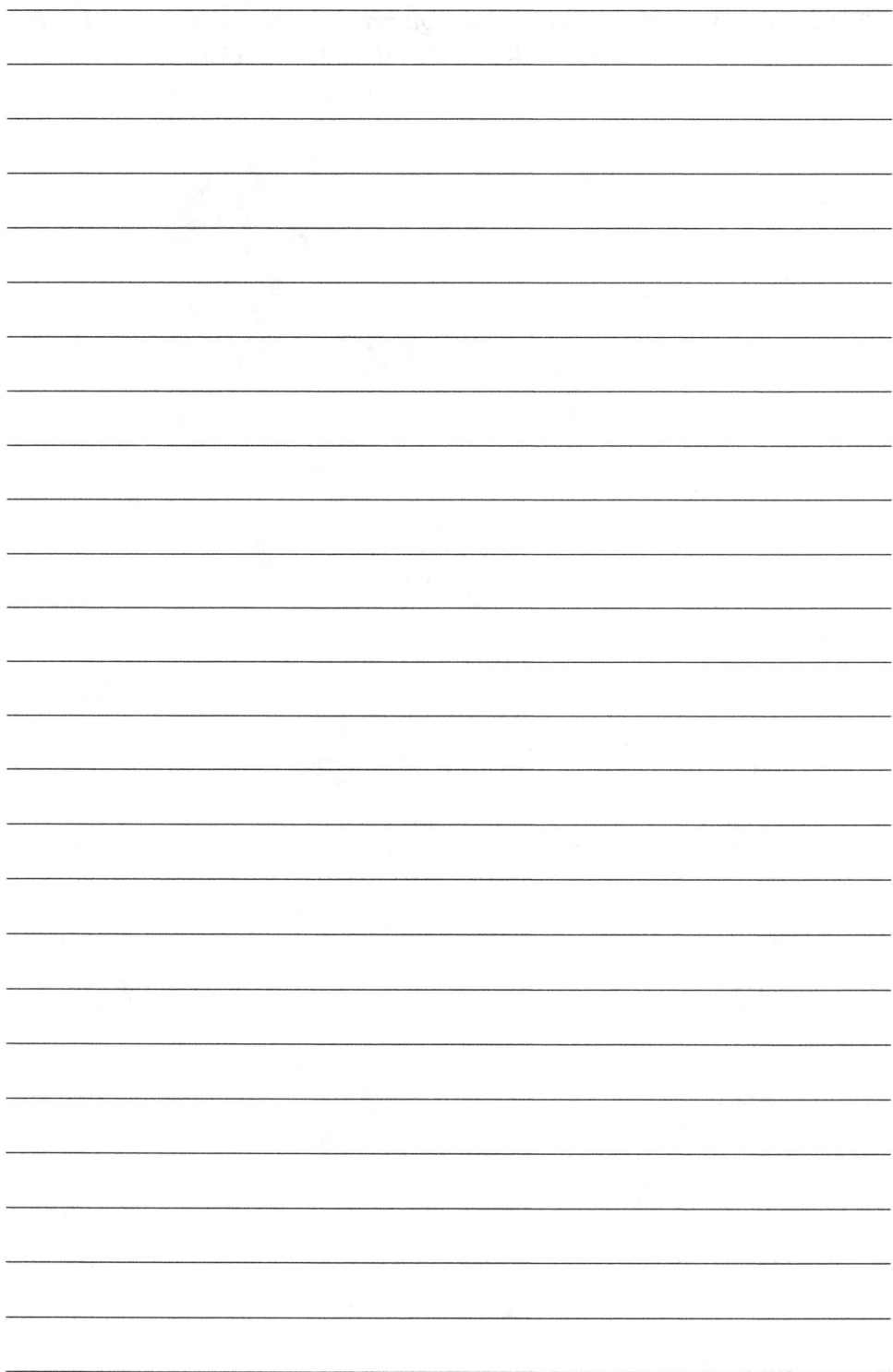

*If food is your best friend, it's also your worst enemy.*

– Edward Jones

_____

_____

_____

_____

_____

_____

_____

_____

_____

_____

_____

_____

_____

_____

_____

_____

_____

_____

_____

_____

_____

_____

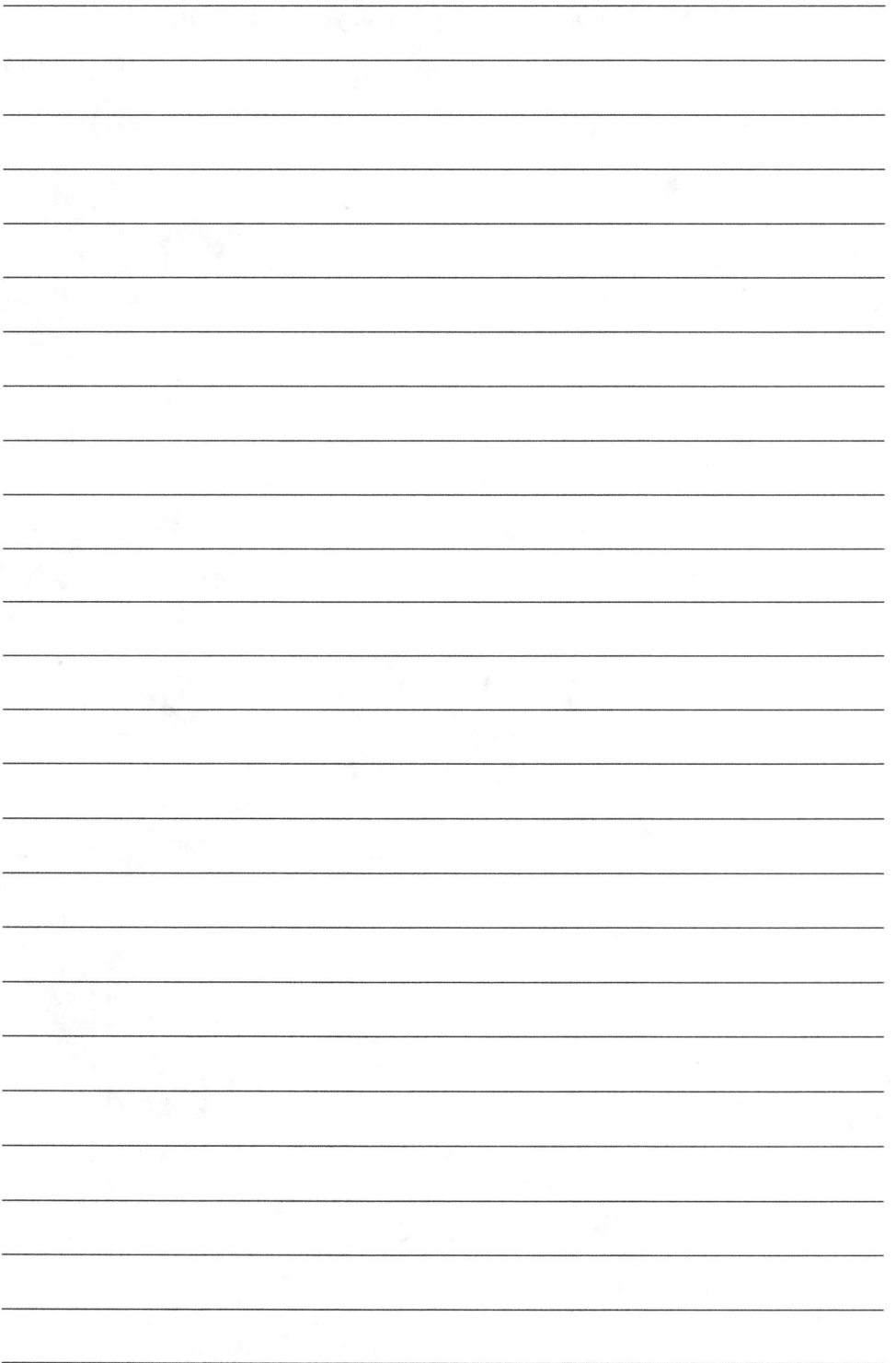

*Make the most of yourself, for that is all there is of you.*

– Ralph Waldo Emerson

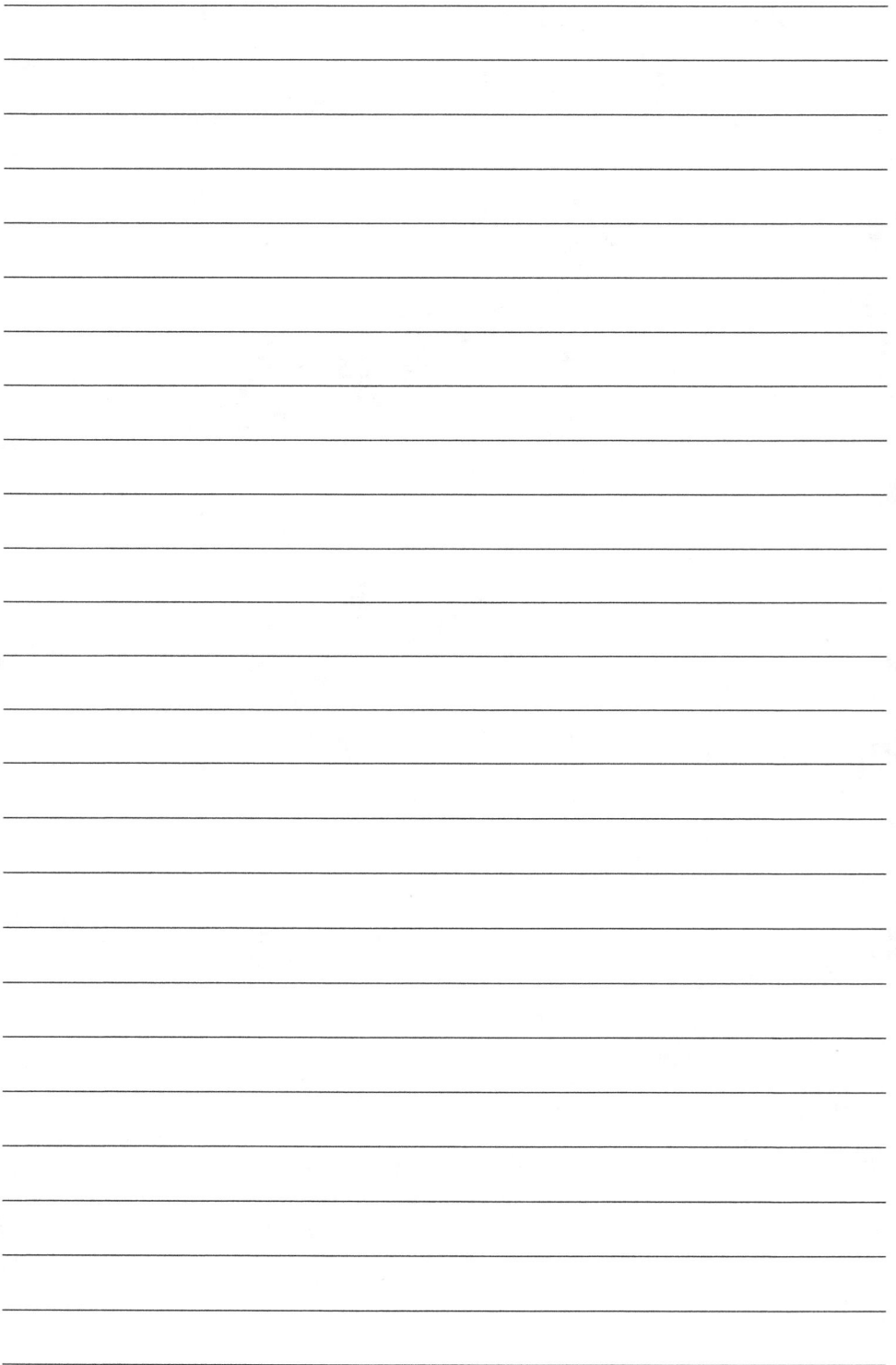

*When you nourish your body with pure energy,*
*you transform from the inside out.*

– Bill Phillips

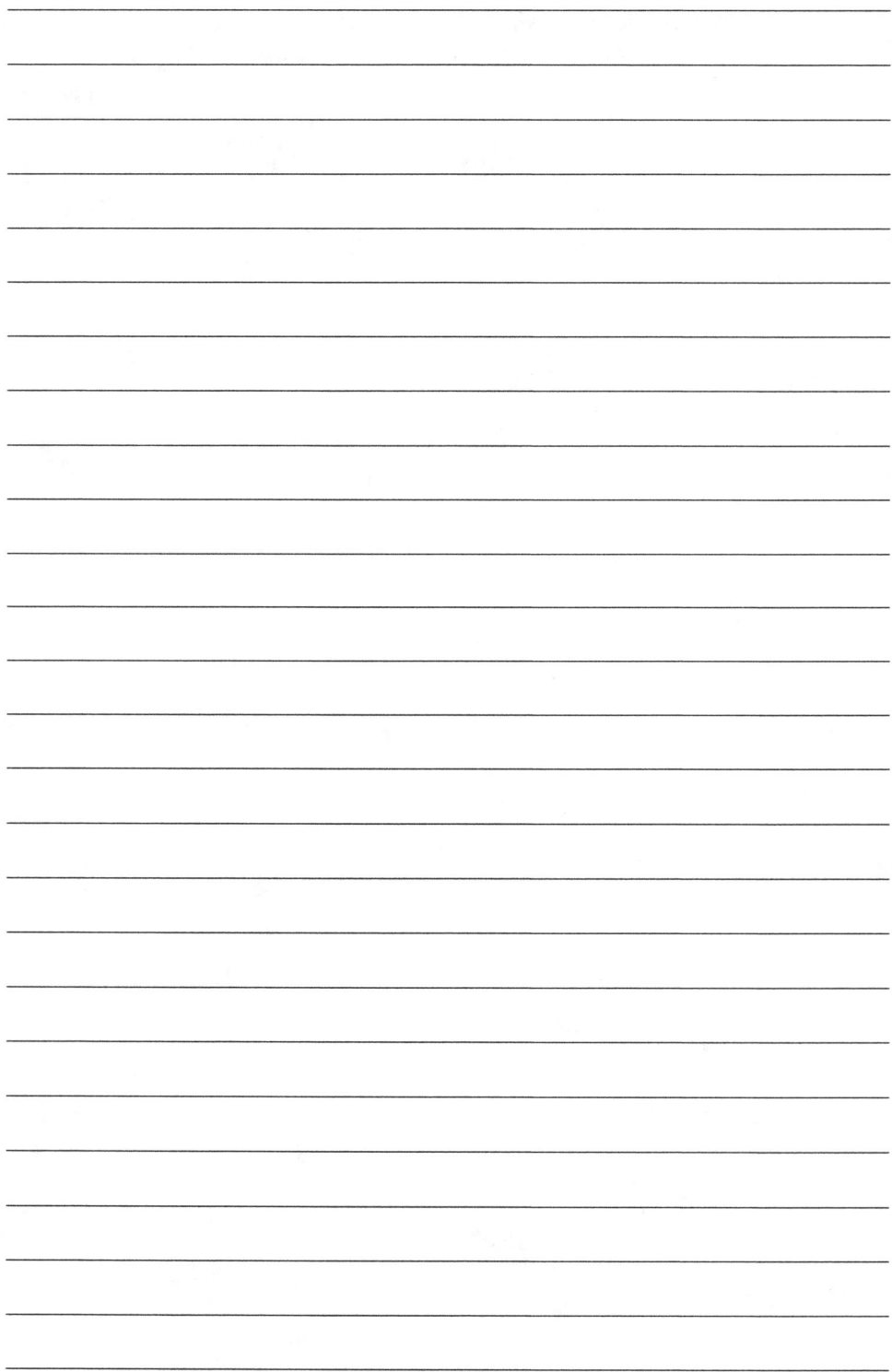

*You don't drown by falling in the water. You drown by staying there.*

– Anonymous

_____

_____

_____

_____

_____

_____

_____

_____

_____

_____

_____

_____

_____

_____

_____

_____

_____

_____

_____

_____

_____

_____

_____

_____

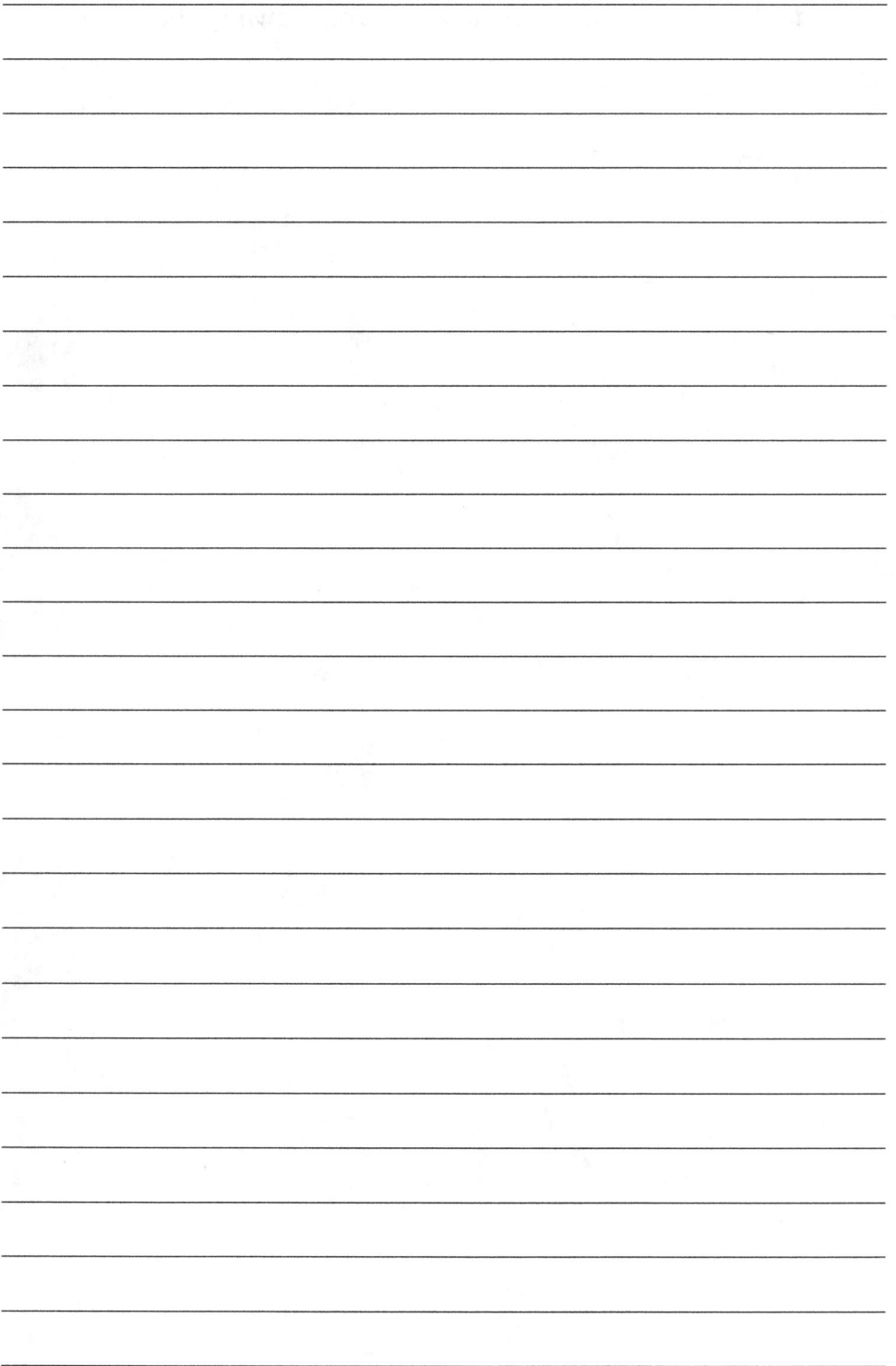

*Tip 10: Practice using the 'healthy plate.' Eat from a 9 inch plate with ½ vegetables and fruit, ¼ heathy grains, and ¼ healthy proteins. Go to* www.choosemyplate.gov *for details*

_____

_____

_____

_____

_____

_____

_____

_____

_____

_____

_____

_____

_____

_____

_____

_____

_____

_____

_____

_____

_____

_____

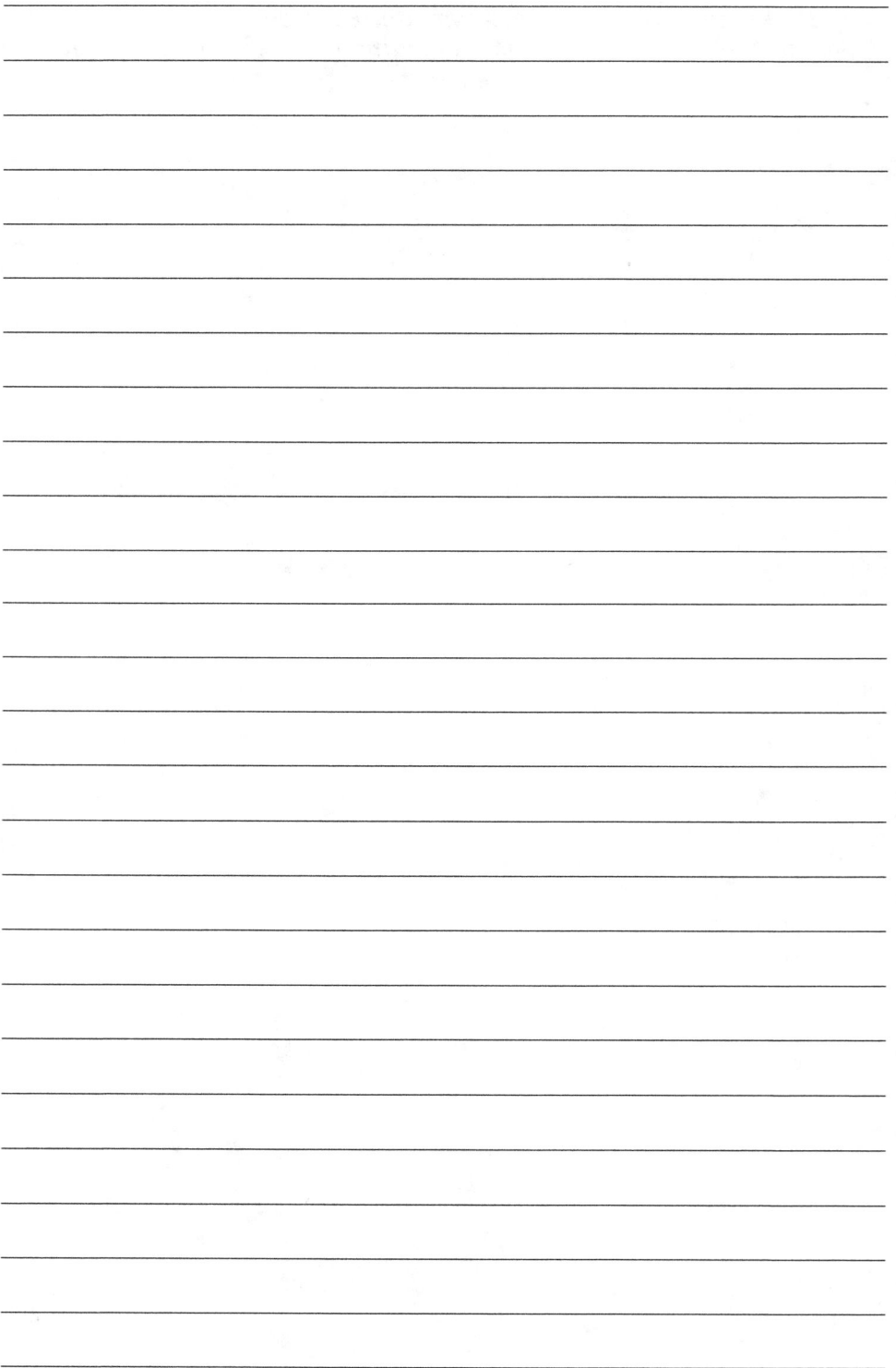

*Take care of your body with steadfast fidelity. The soul must see through these eyes alone, and if they are dim, the whole world is clouded.*

– Goethe

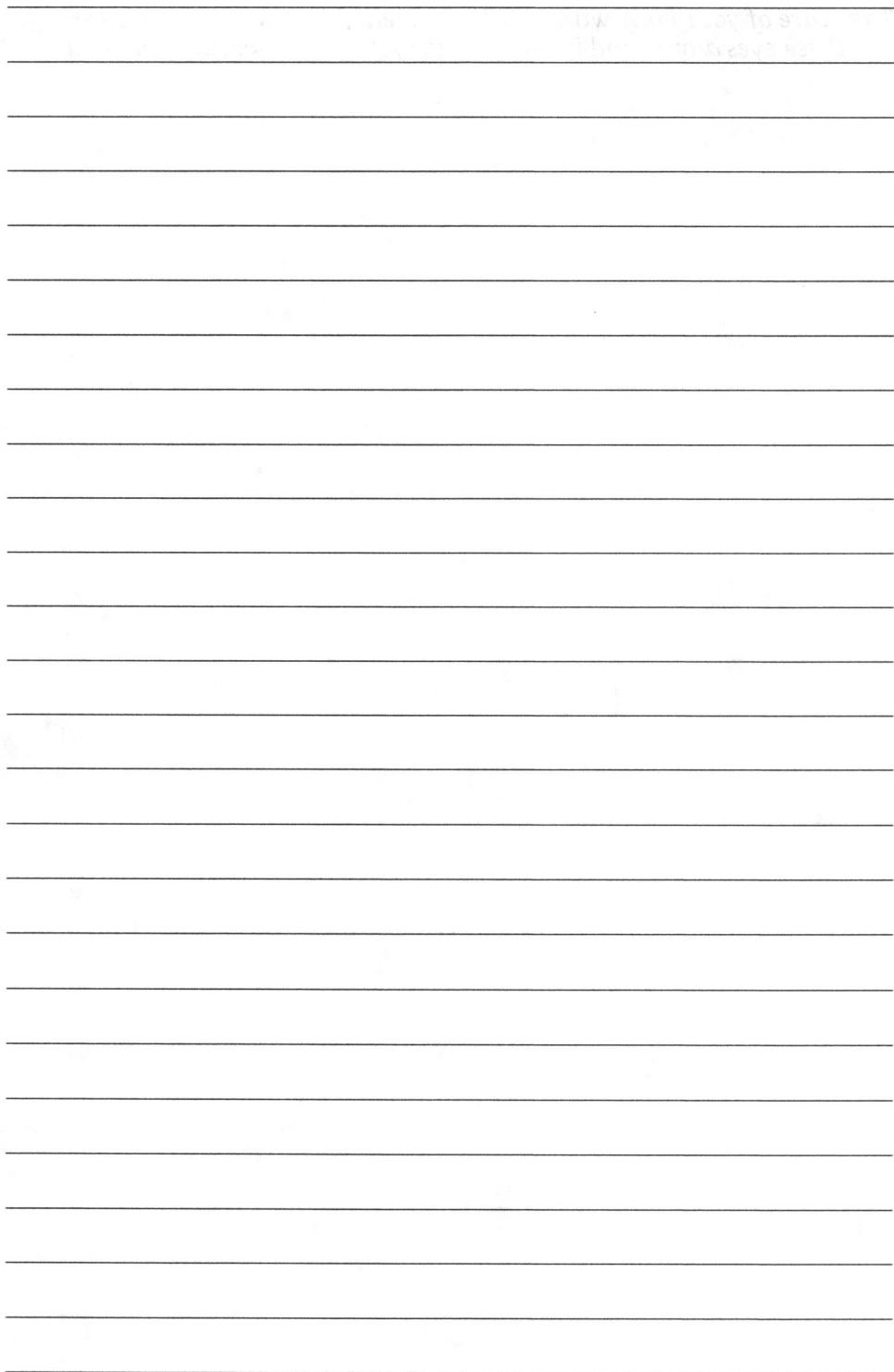

*We can reverse years of damage to our bodies by deciding to raise our standards for ourselves, then living differently. Old wounds heal, injuries repair, and the whole system improves with just a few changes in what we put into our bodies and how we move them.*

– Anonymous

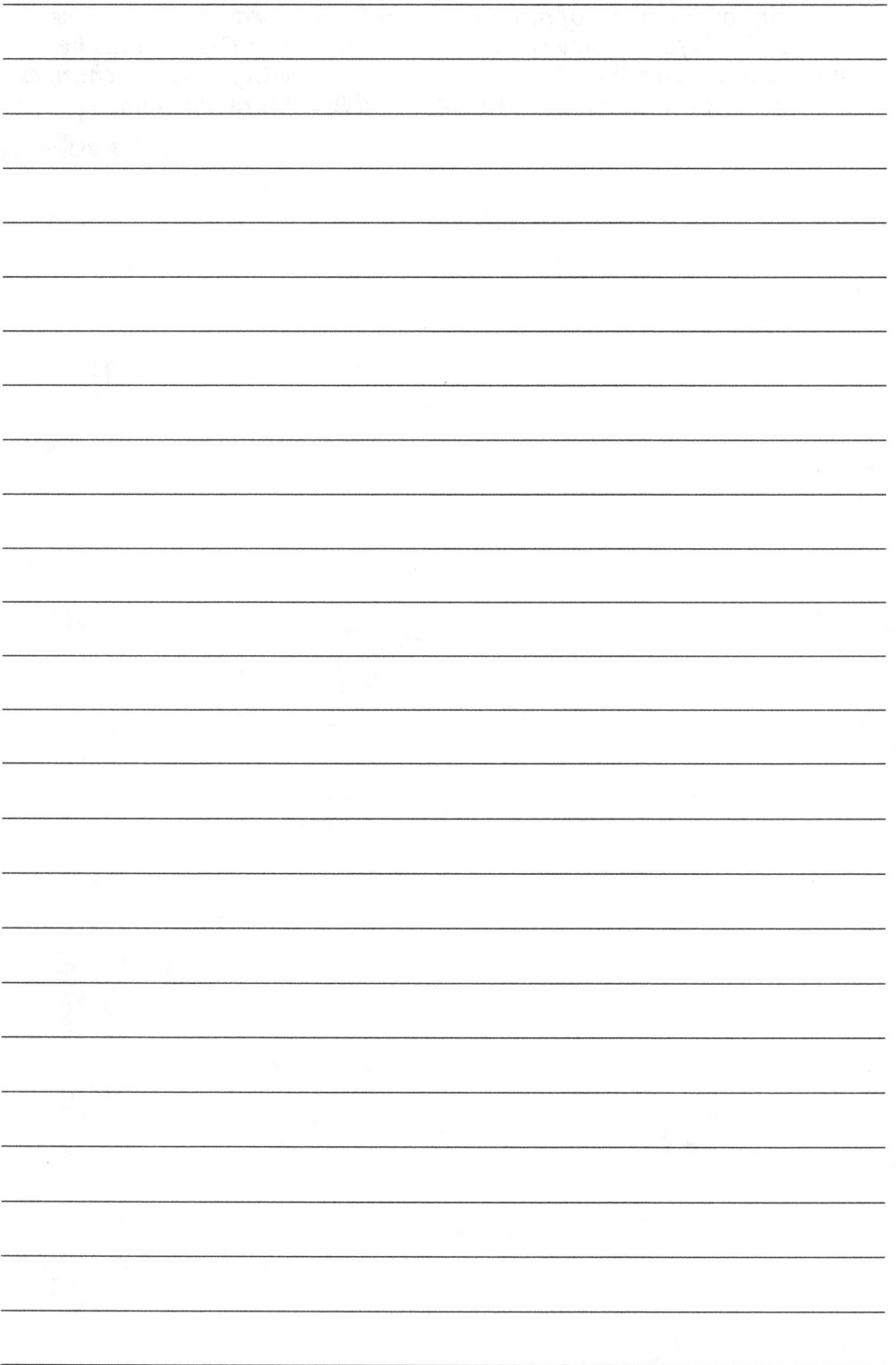

*Tip 11: BMI is used to determine obesity. It is calculated by dividing your weight in kilograms by your height in meters squared.*

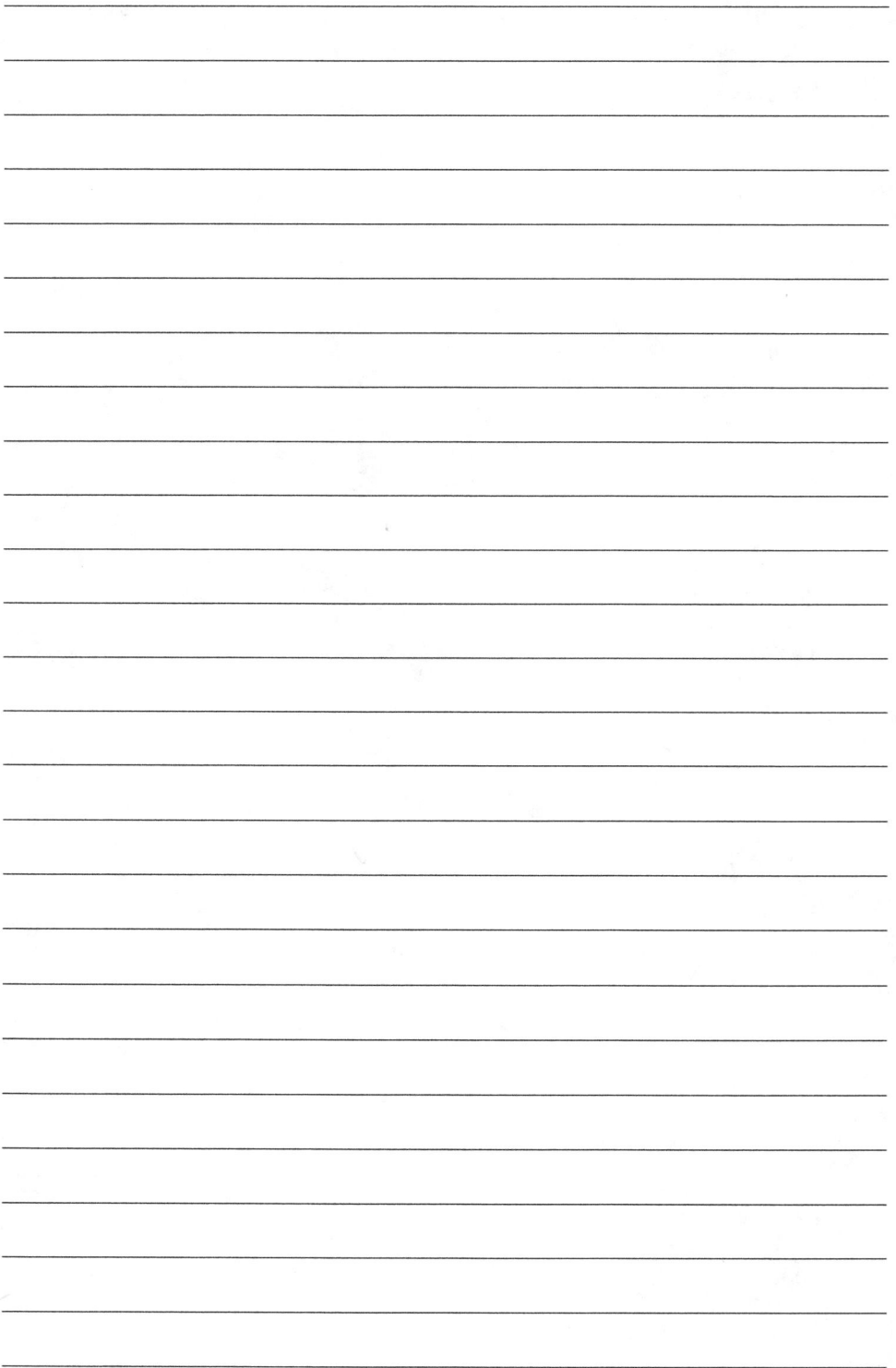

*Love is the great miracle cure.*
*Loving ourselves works miracles in our lives.*

– Louise Hay, Cancer survivor

_____

_____

_____

_____

_____

_____

_____

_____

_____

_____

_____

_____

_____

_____

_____

_____

_____

_____

_____

_____

_____

_____

_____

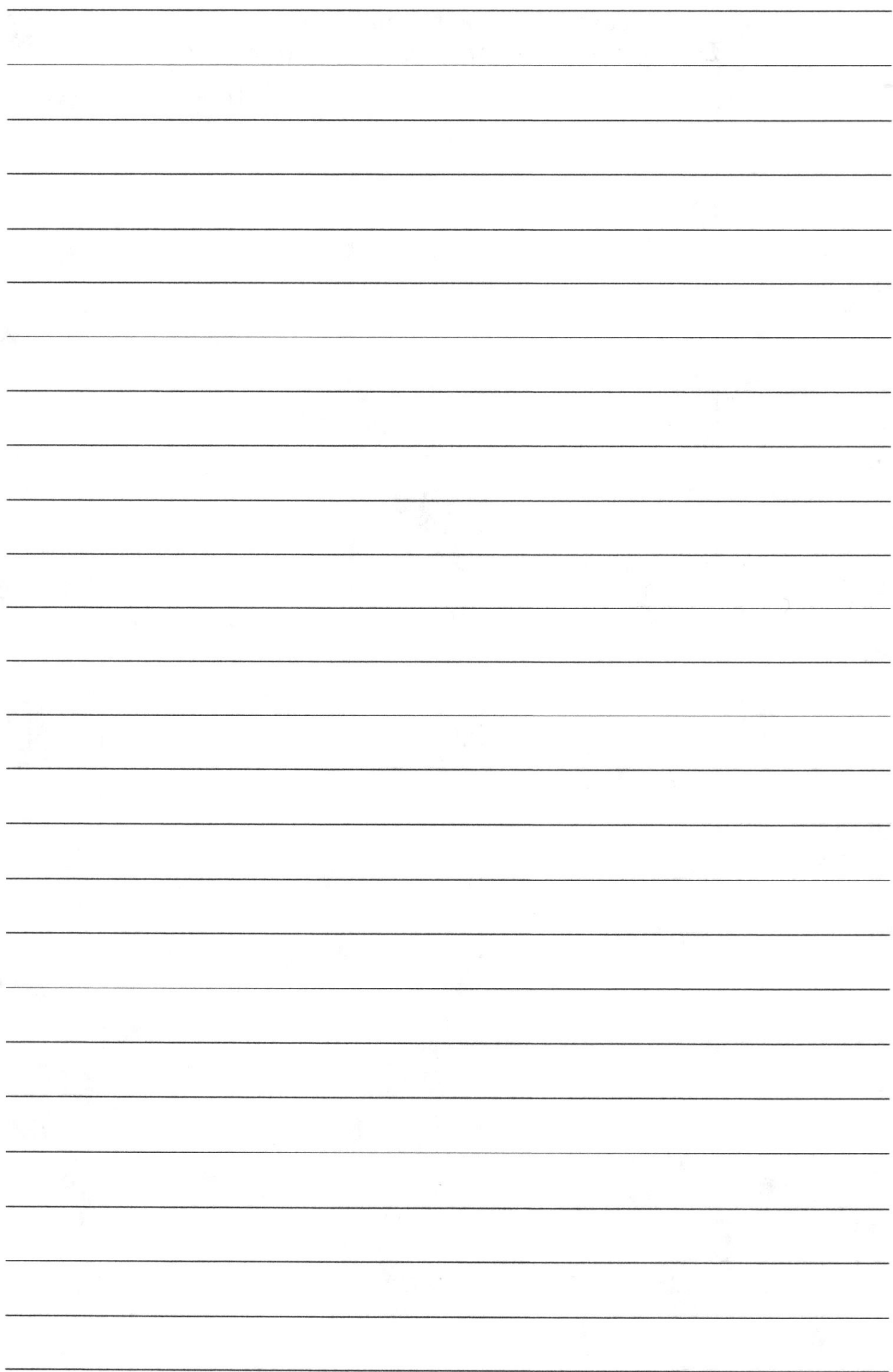

*The physical world, including our bodies, is a response of the observer.*
*We create our bodies as we create the experience of our world.*

– Dr. Deepak Chopra

_____

_____

_____

_____

_____

_____

_____

_____

_____

_____

_____

_____

_____

_____

_____

_____

_____

_____

_____

_____

_____

_____

_____

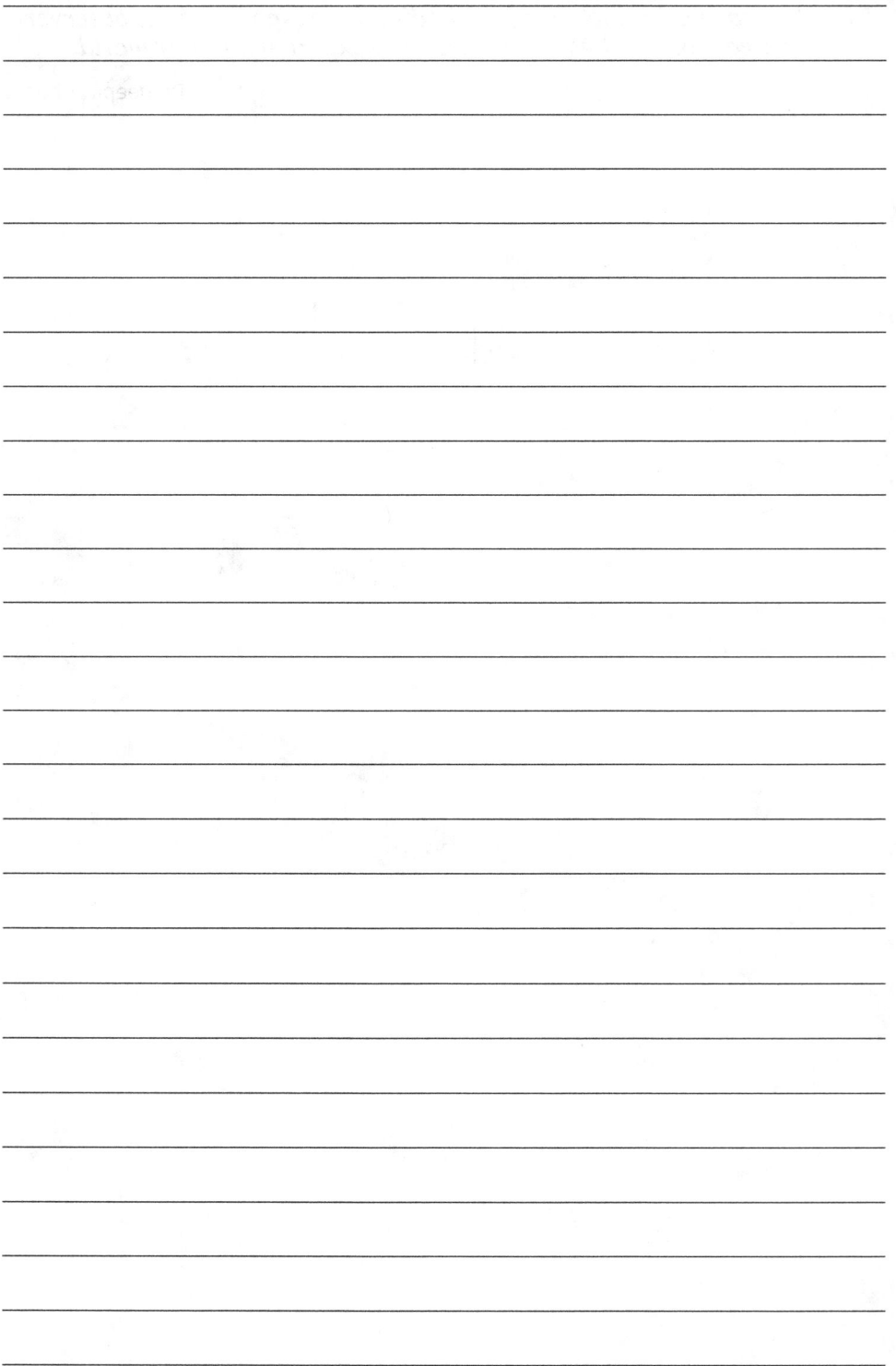

*Tip 12: BMI Category - Underweight is < 18.5, Normal is 18.5- 24.9,*
*Overweight 25-29.9, Obesity 30-39.9, Severe obesity > 40.*
*Calculate your BMI to see how much you need to lose. BMI Calculator*
https://www.nhlbi.nih.gov/health/educational/lose_wt/BMI/bmicalc.htm

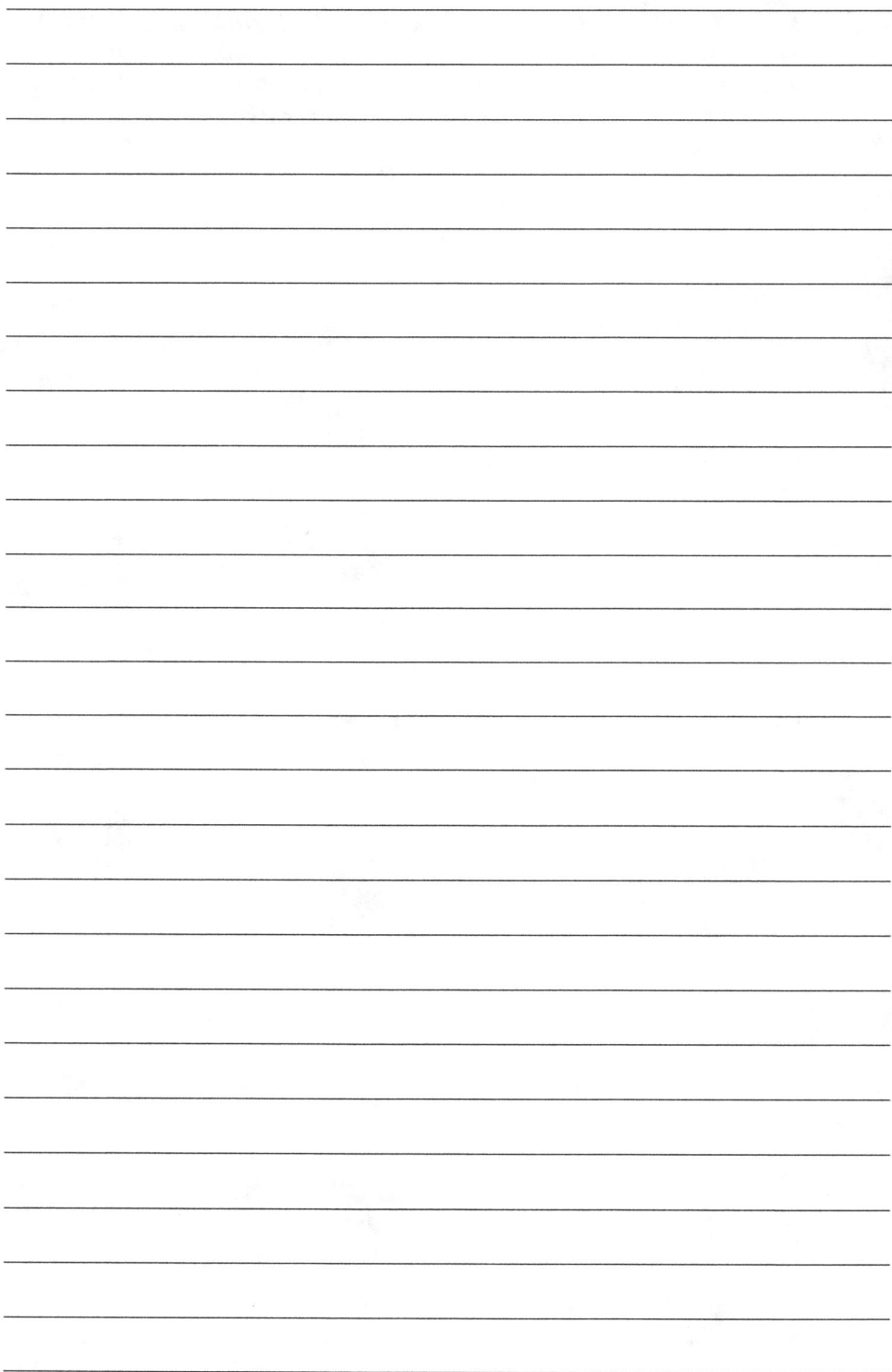

*The cell is immortal. It is merely the fluid in which it floats that degenerates. Renew this fluid at regular intervals, give the cells what they require for nutrition, and as far as we know, the pulsation of life can go on forever.*

– Dr. Alexis Carrell, <small>Nobel prize winner</small>

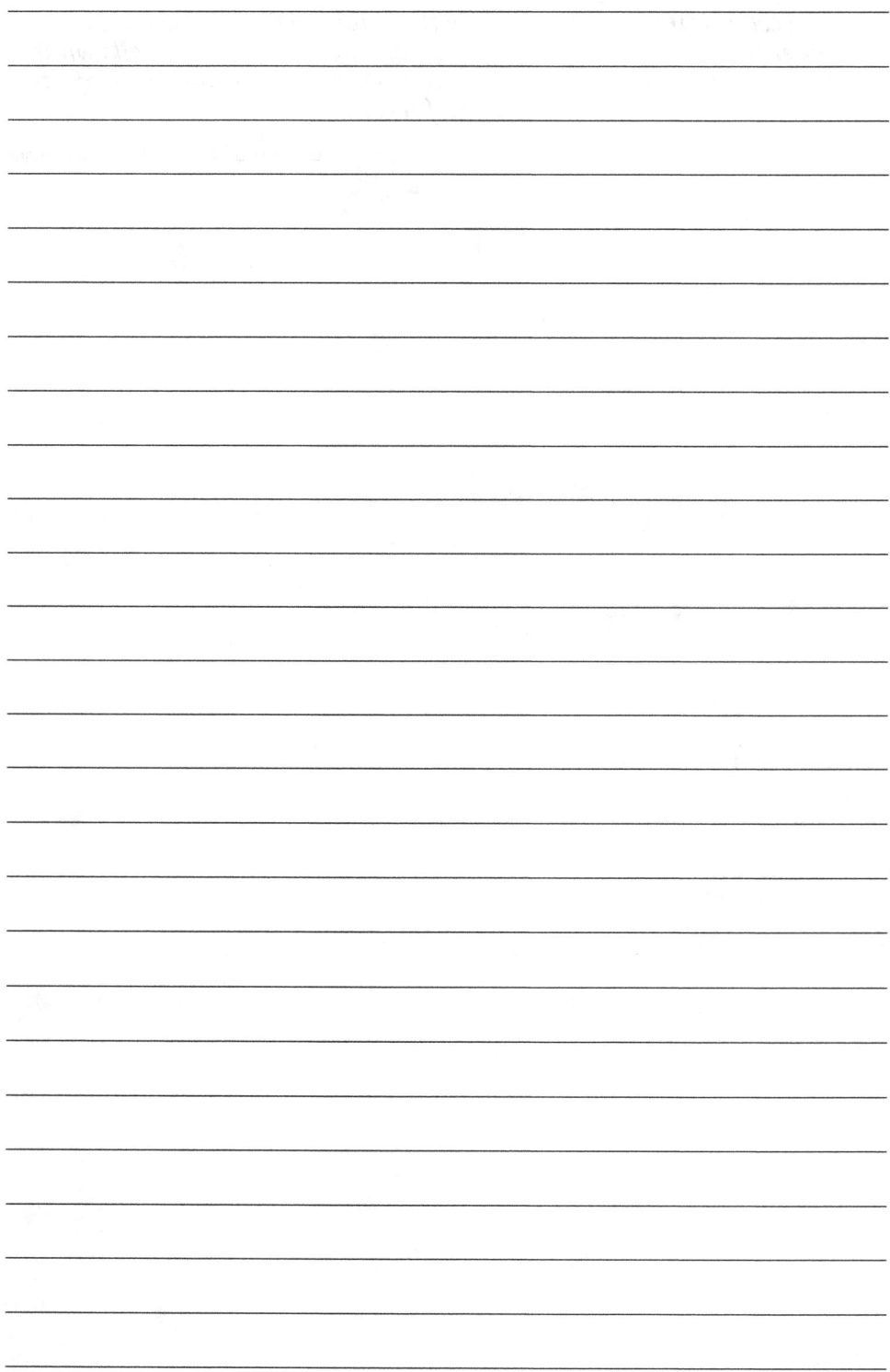

*The human body heals itself and nutrition provides*
*the resources to accomplish the task.*

– Roger Williams Ph.D.

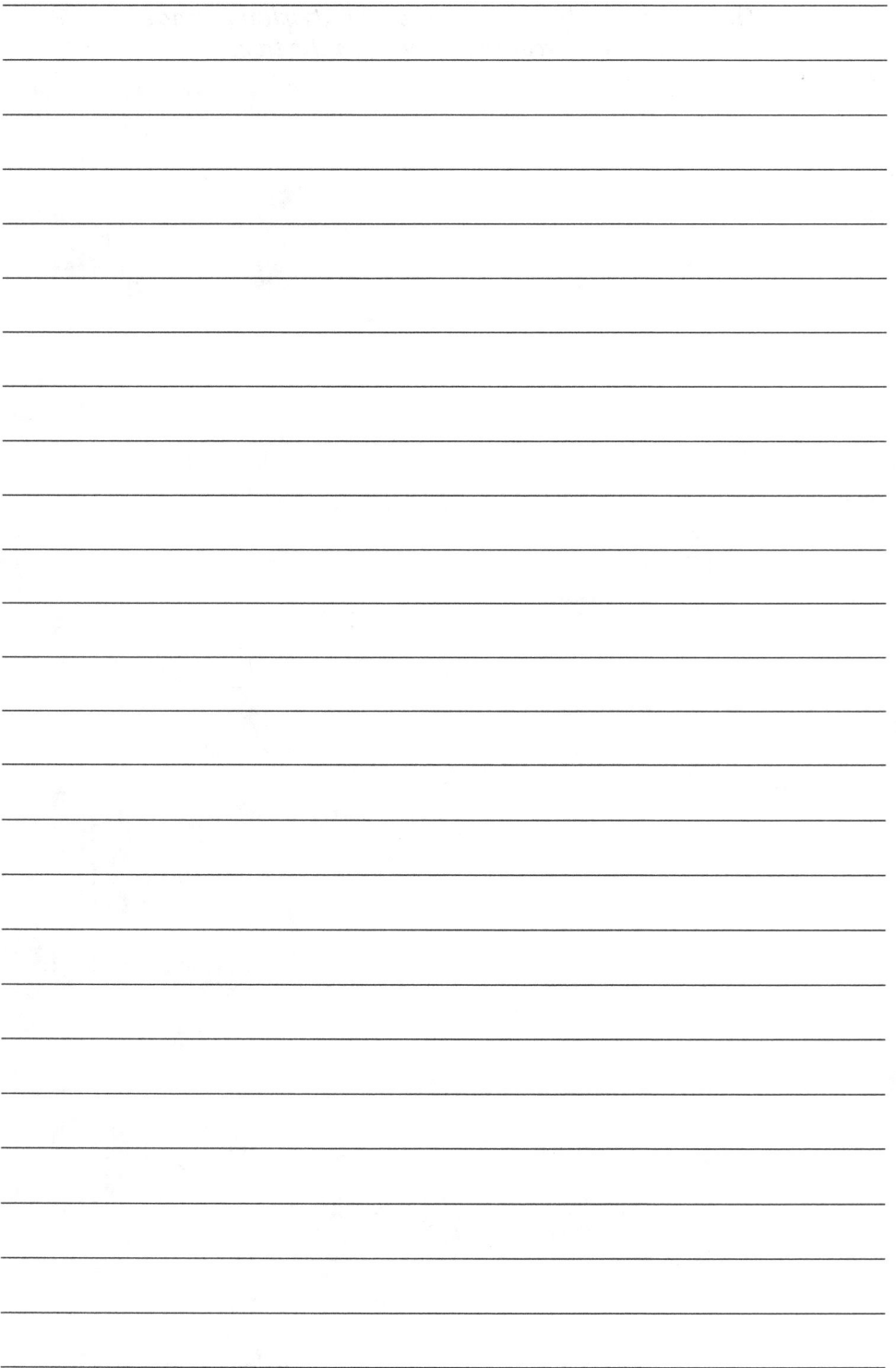

*There's something called the physiology of forgiveness. Being unable to forgive other people's faults is harmful to one's health.*

– Dr. Herbert Benson

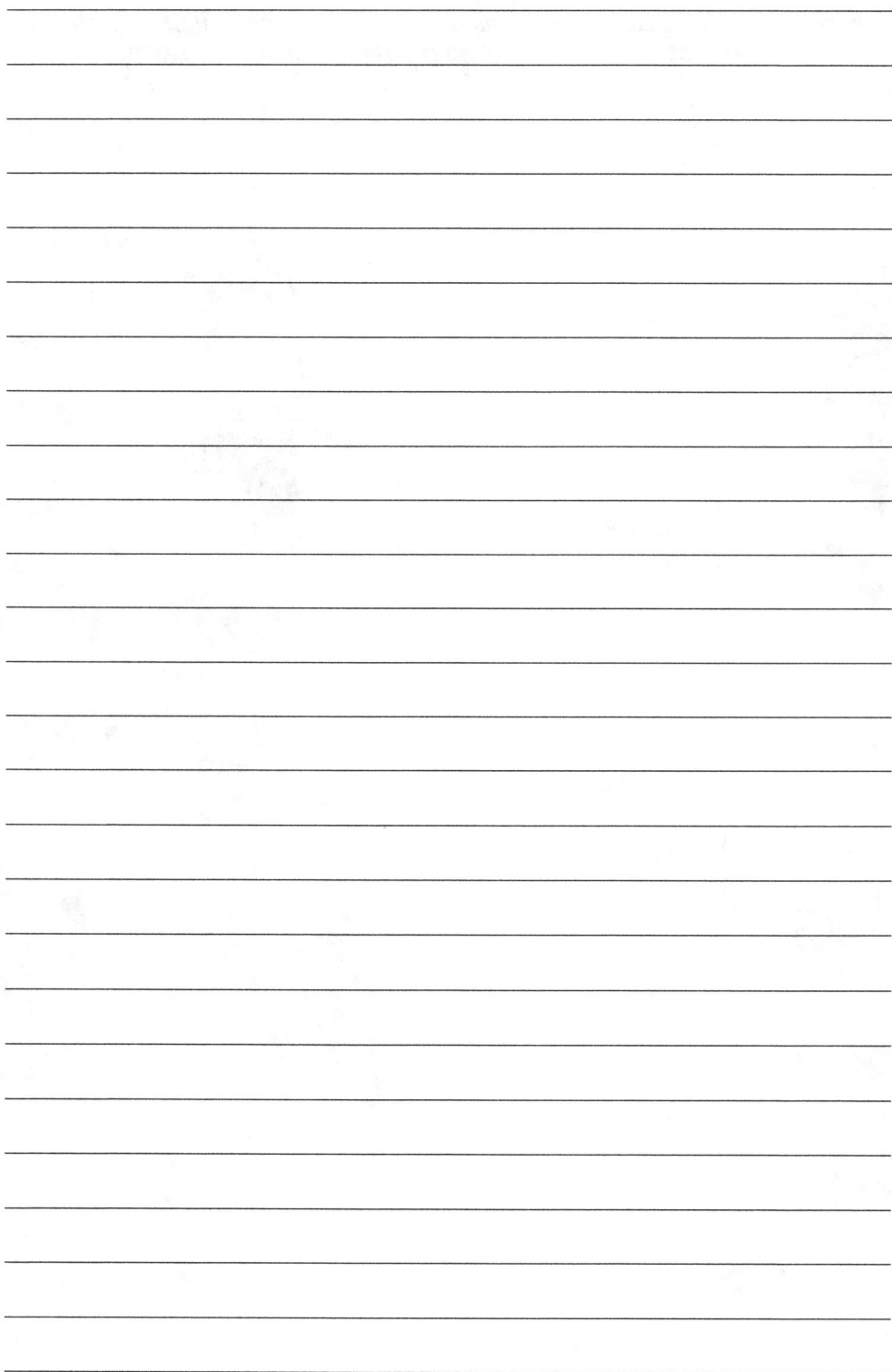

*Tip 13: Chew slowly. This gives your brain a chance to realize that you are full. Chewing slowly has been associated with lower calorie intake.*

_____

_____

_____

_____

_____

_____

_____

_____

_____

_____

_____

_____

_____

_____

_____

_____

_____

_____

_____

_____

_____

_____

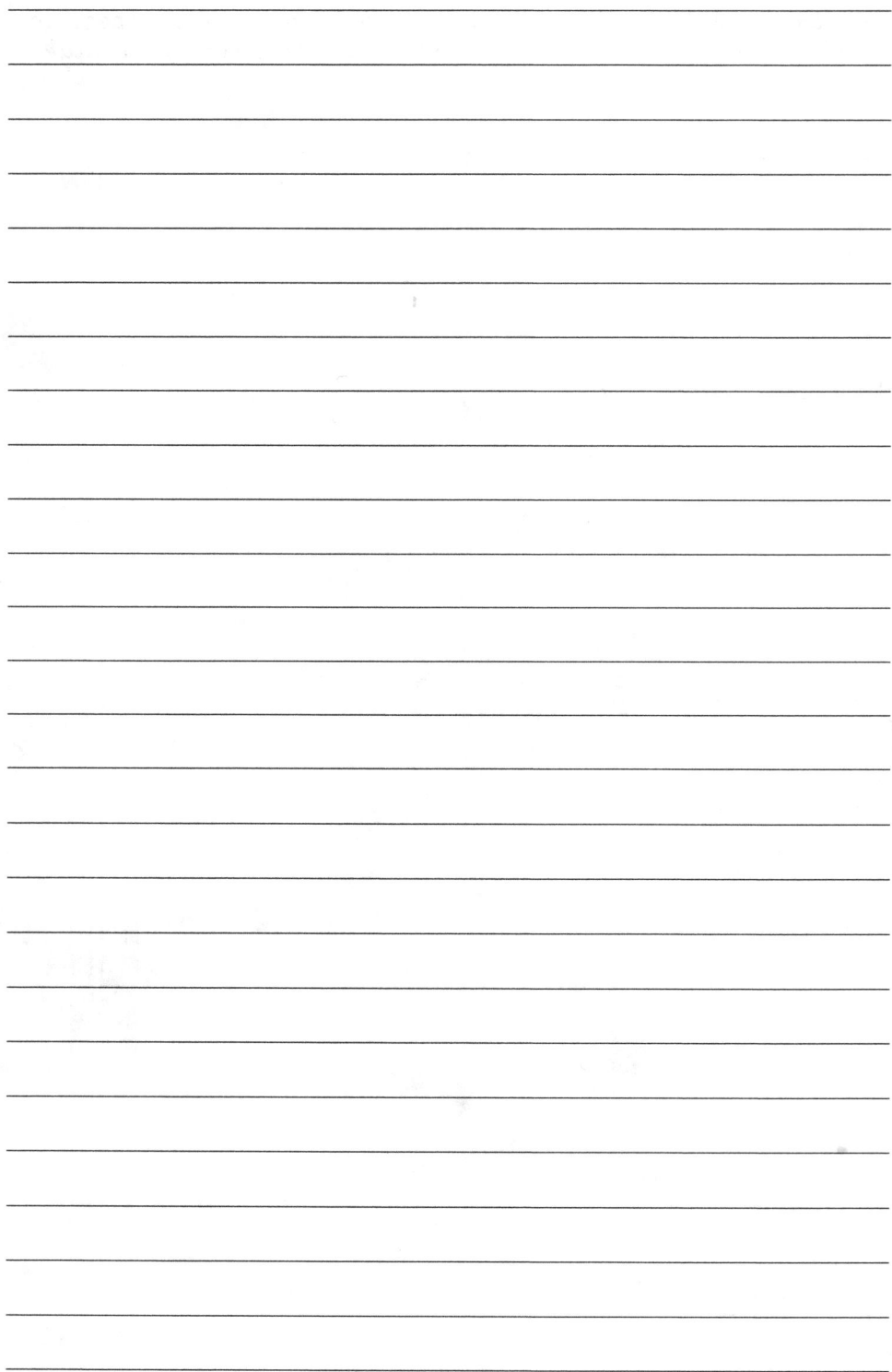

*If you keep on eating unhealthy food then no matter how many weight loss tips you follow, you are likely to retain weight and become obese. If only you start eating healthy food, you will be pleasantly surprised how easy it is to lose weight.*

– Subodh Gupta, 7 habits of skinny woman

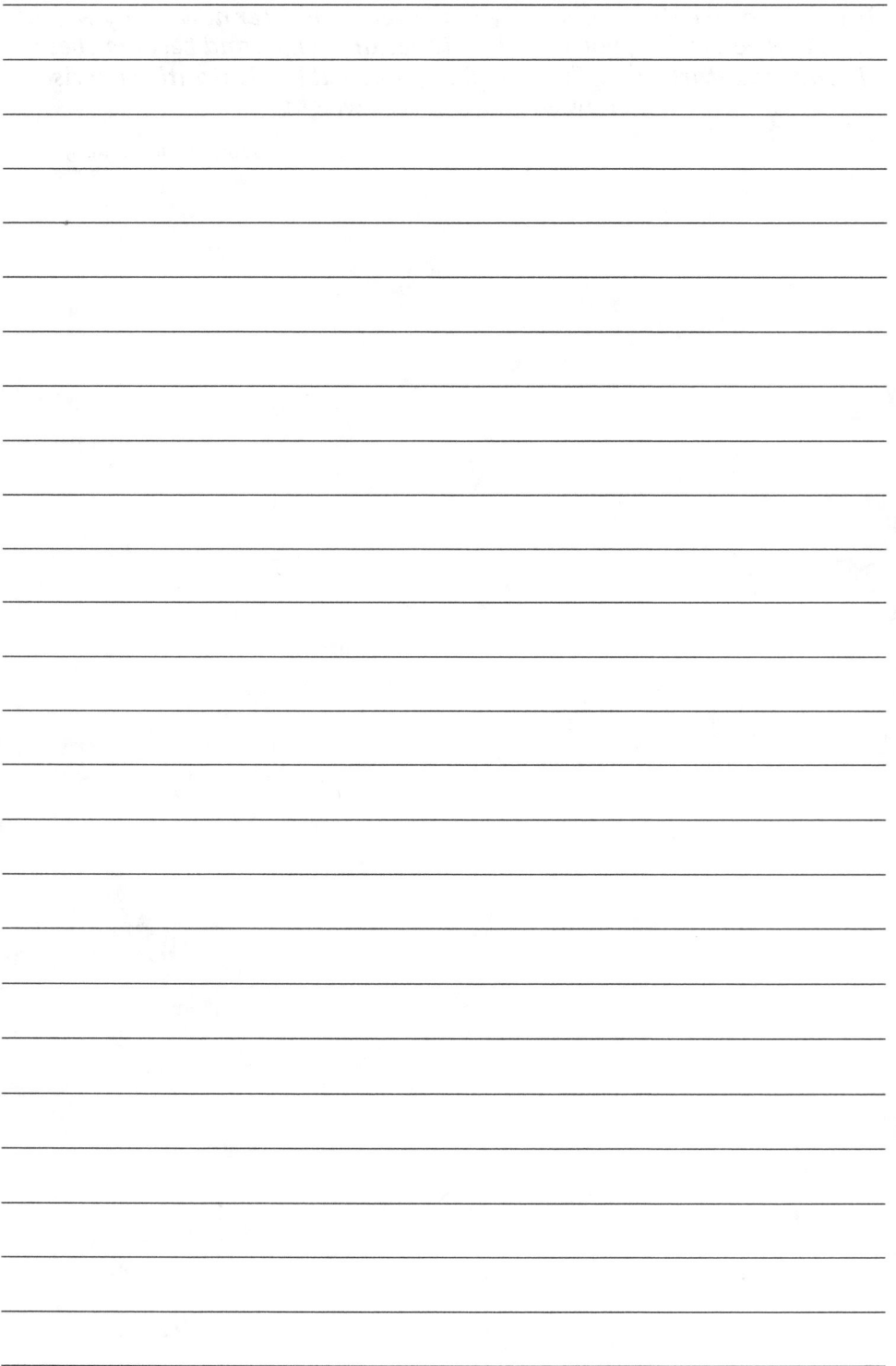

*If I'd known I was going to live this long,*
*I'd have taken better care of myself.*

– Eubie Blake

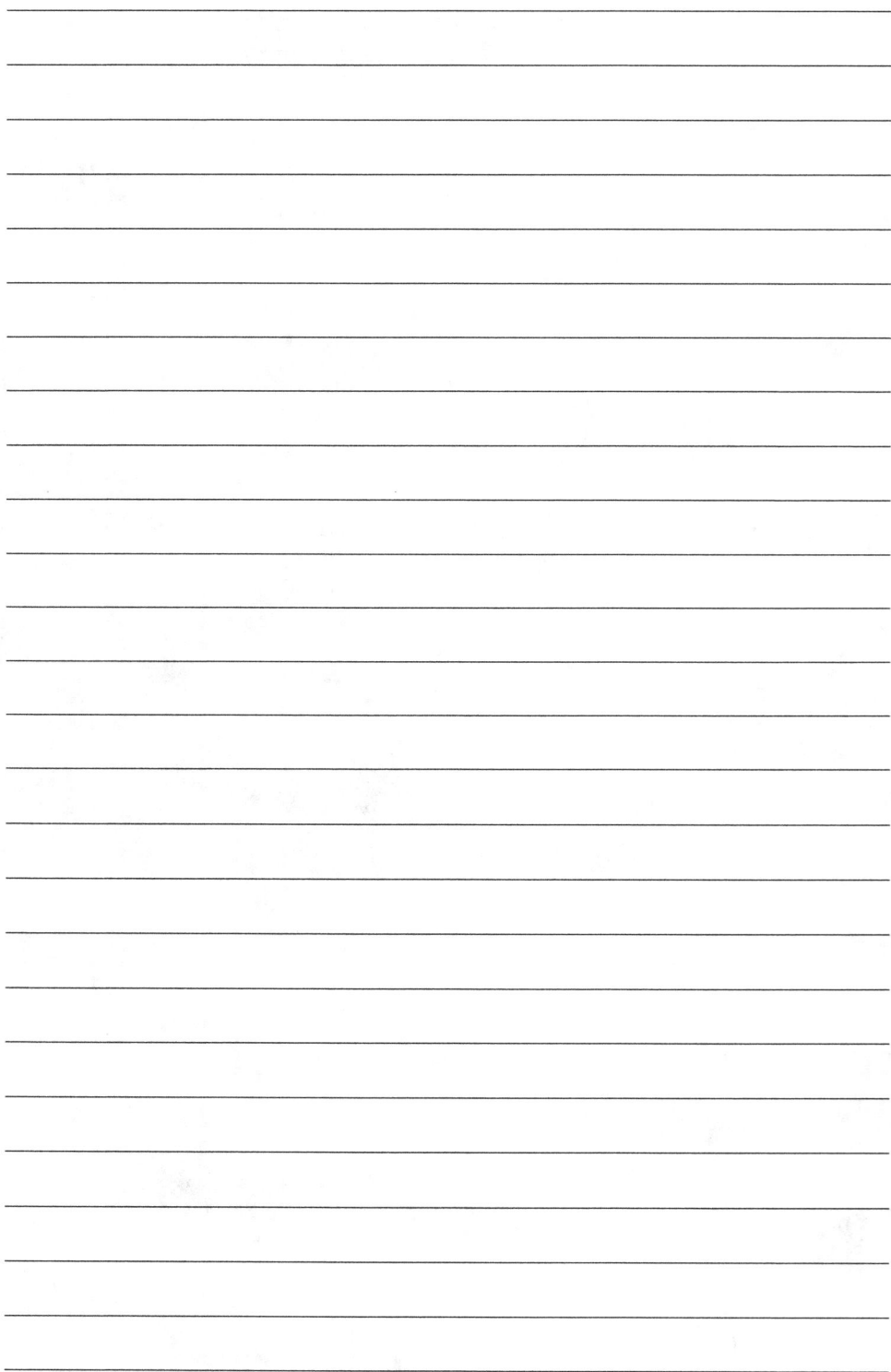

*Every human being is the author of his own health or disease.*

– Buddha

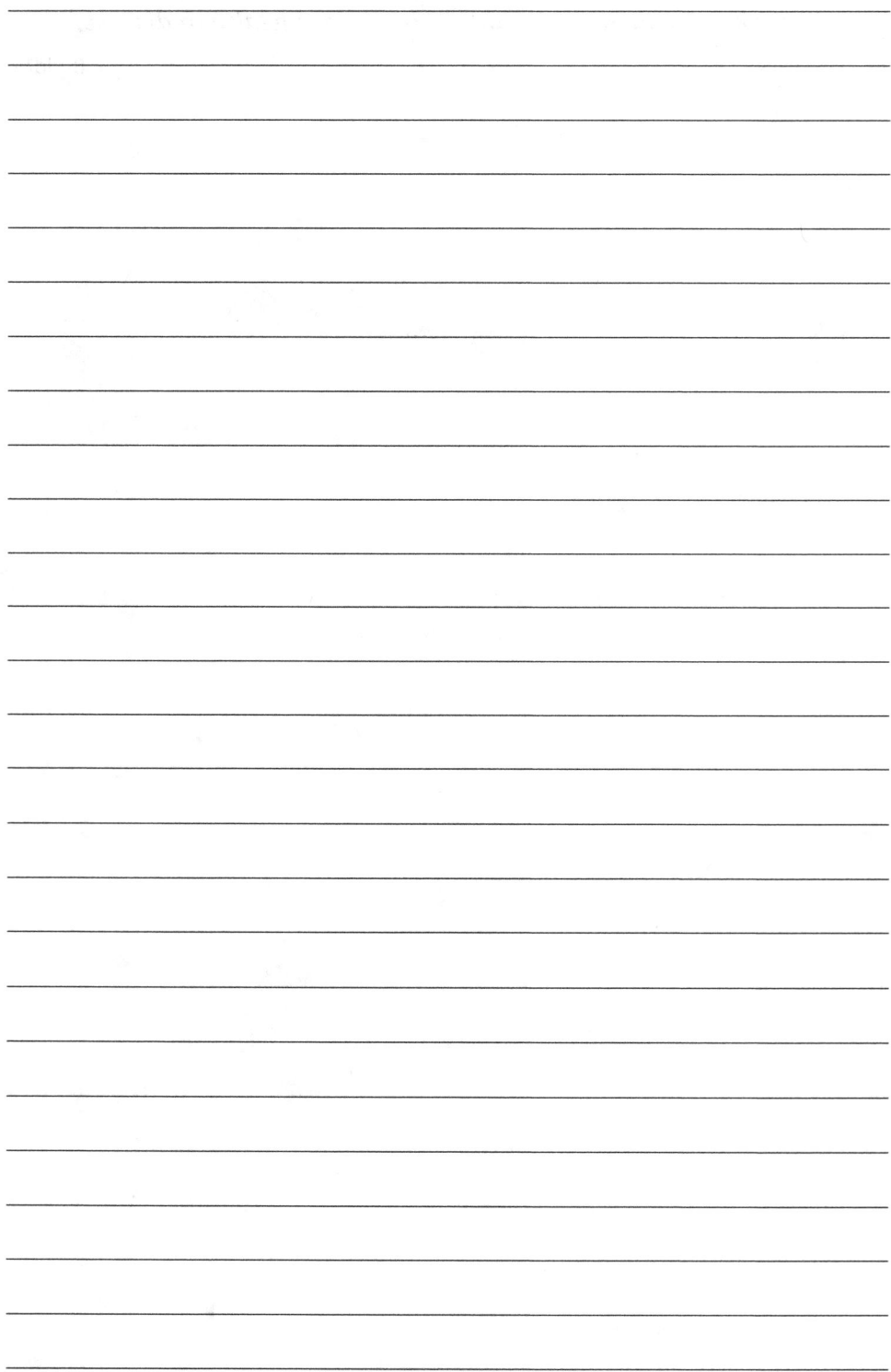

*Bigger snacks mean bigger slacks.*

– Unknown

_____

_____

_____

_____

_____

_____

_____

_____

_____

_____

_____

_____

_____

_____

_____

_____

_____

_____

_____

_____

_____

_____

_____

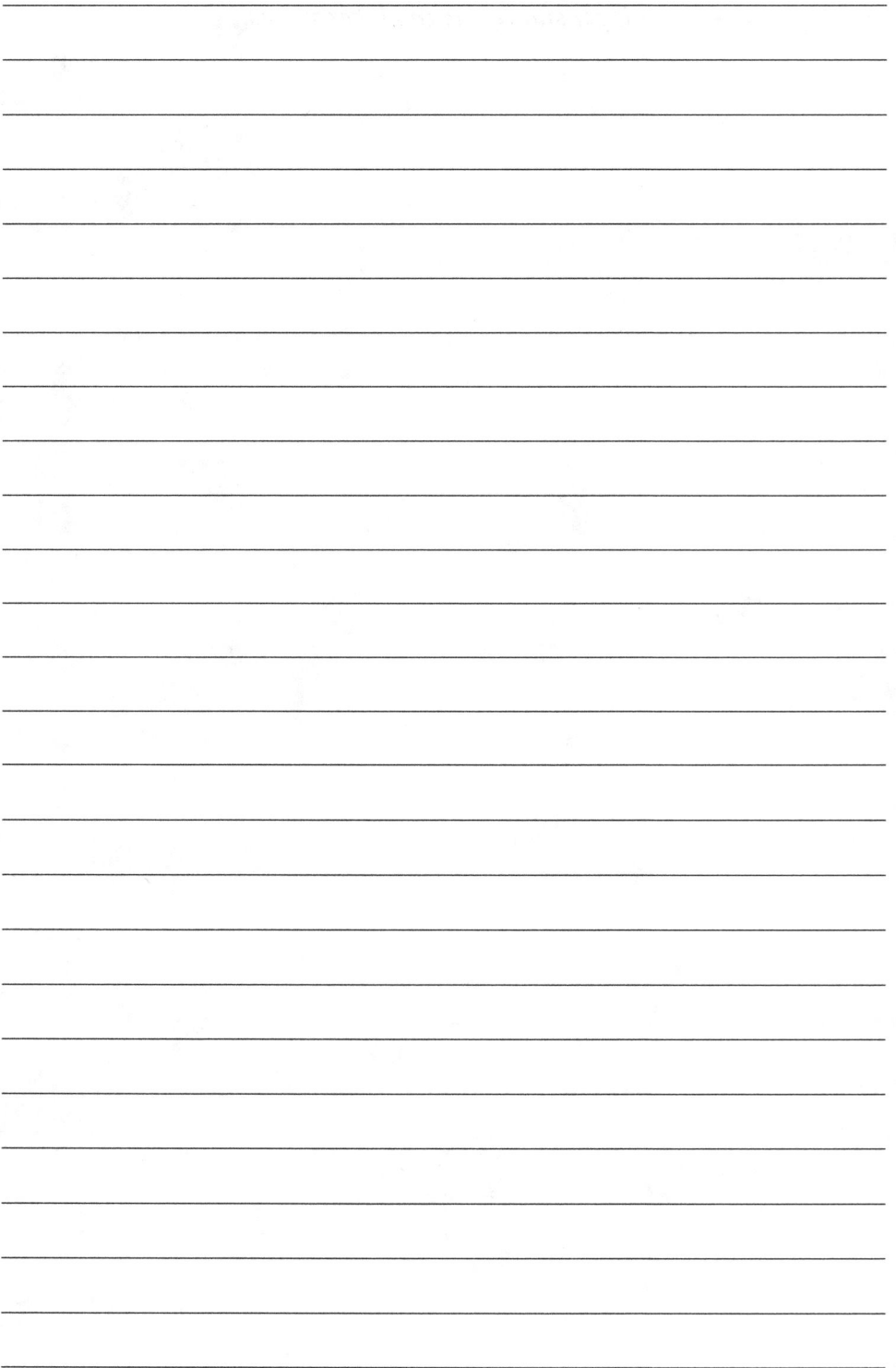

*Tip 14: Avoid sugary beverages. Drinks such as soda and juices are simply sugar and water with very little nutrients. If you like the fizz associated with soda, drink seltzer water instead.*

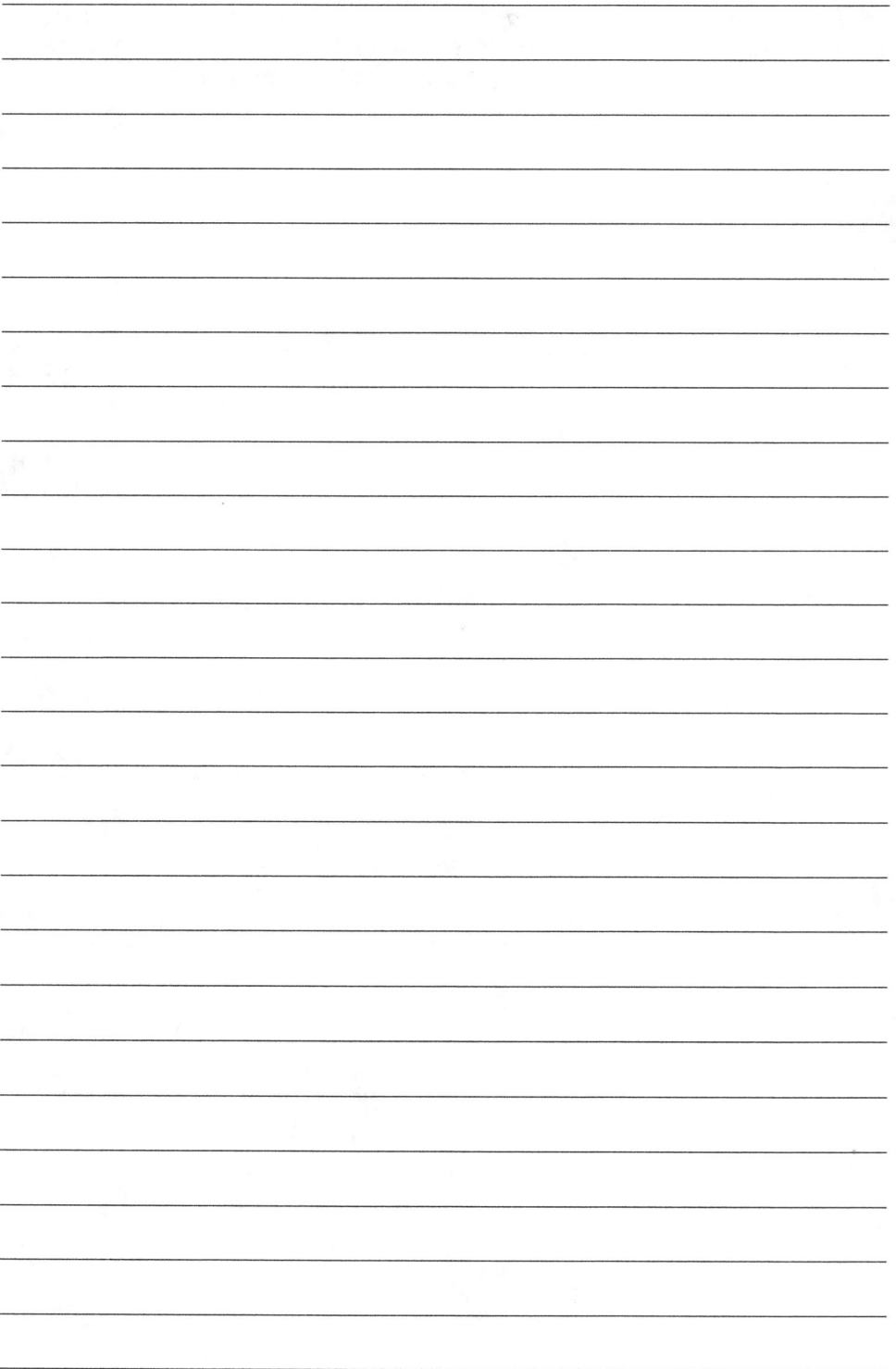

*What you eat in private will show up in public.*

– Unknown

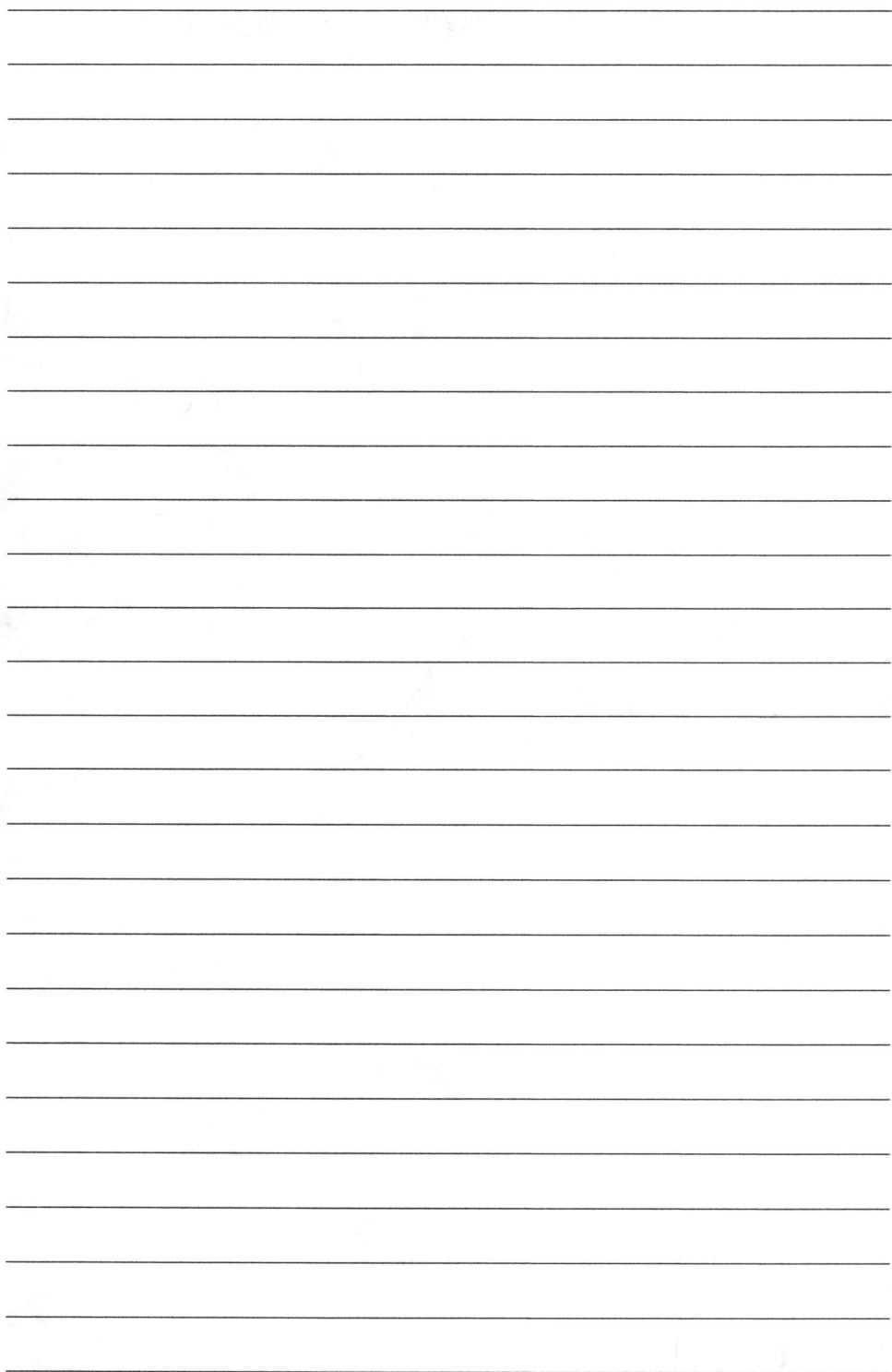

*Don't dig your grave with your own knife and fork.*

– English Proverb

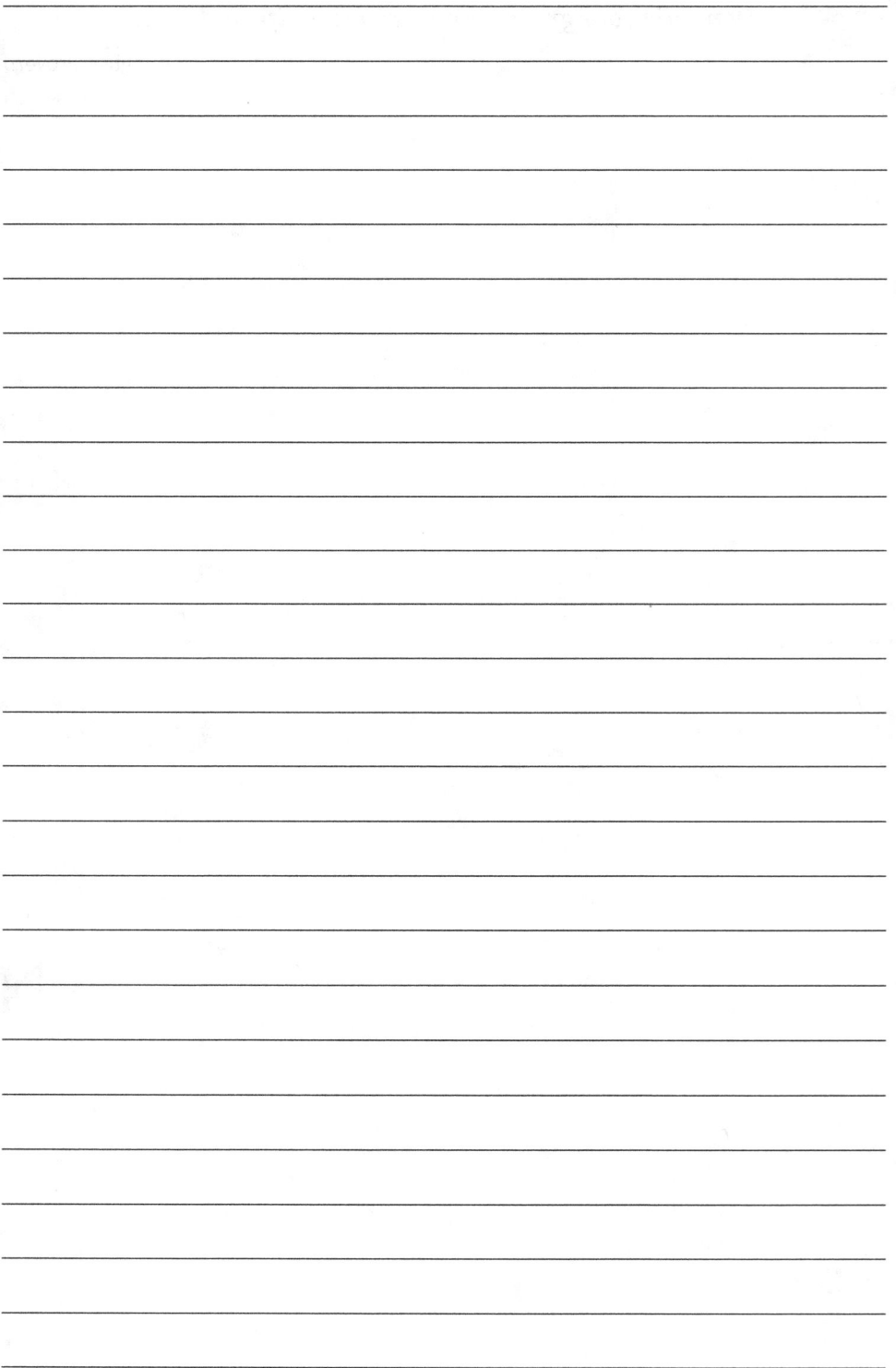

*Time And health are two precious assets that we don't recognize and appreciate until they have been depleted.*

– Denis Waitley

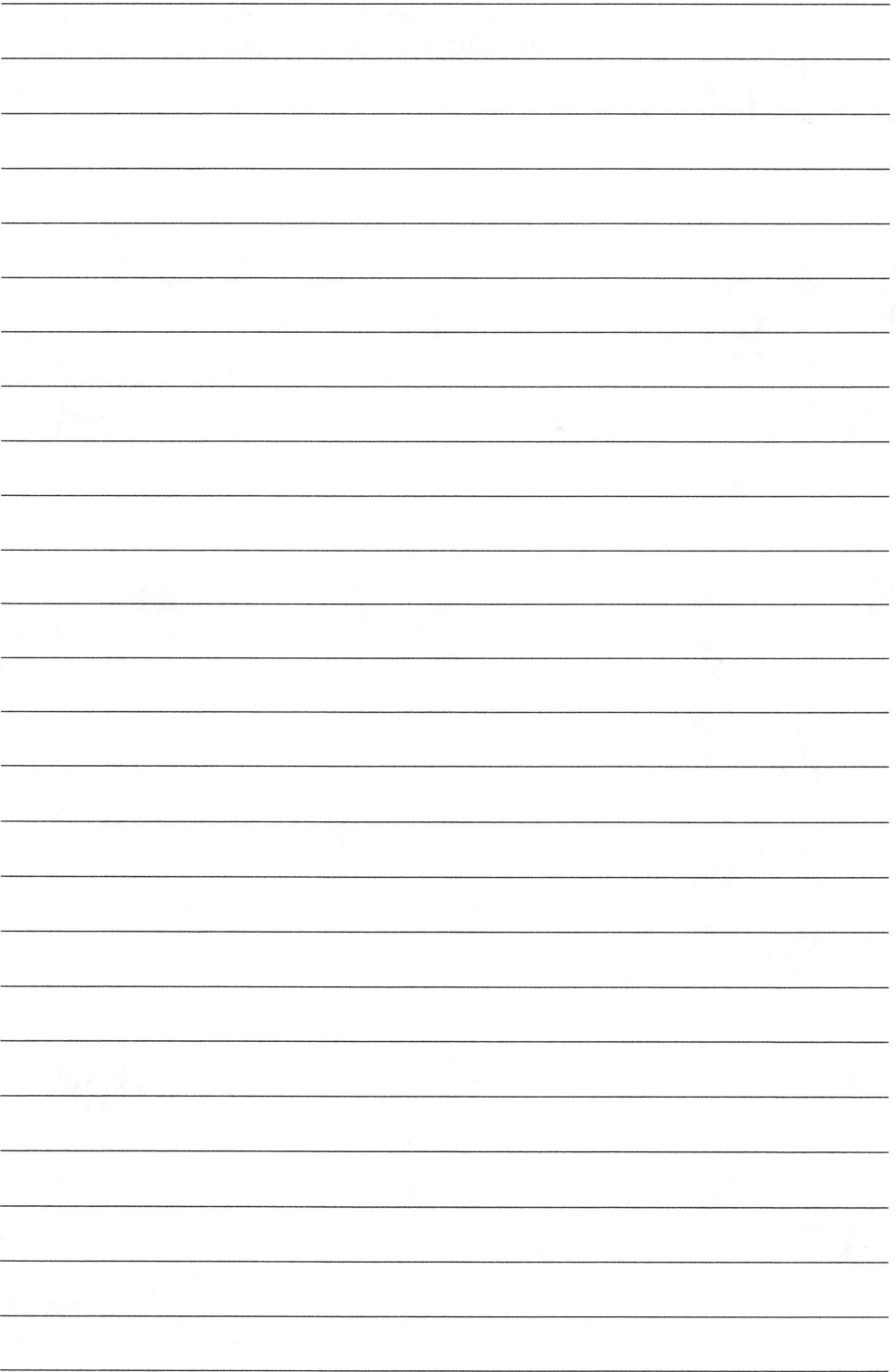

*Tip 15: Avoid going on diets and chose to healthy lifestyle instead. Diets often don't last, and yoyo dieting is bad for your health.*

_____

_____

_____

_____

_____

_____

_____

_____

_____

_____

_____

_____

_____

_____

_____

_____

_____

_____

_____

_____

_____

_____

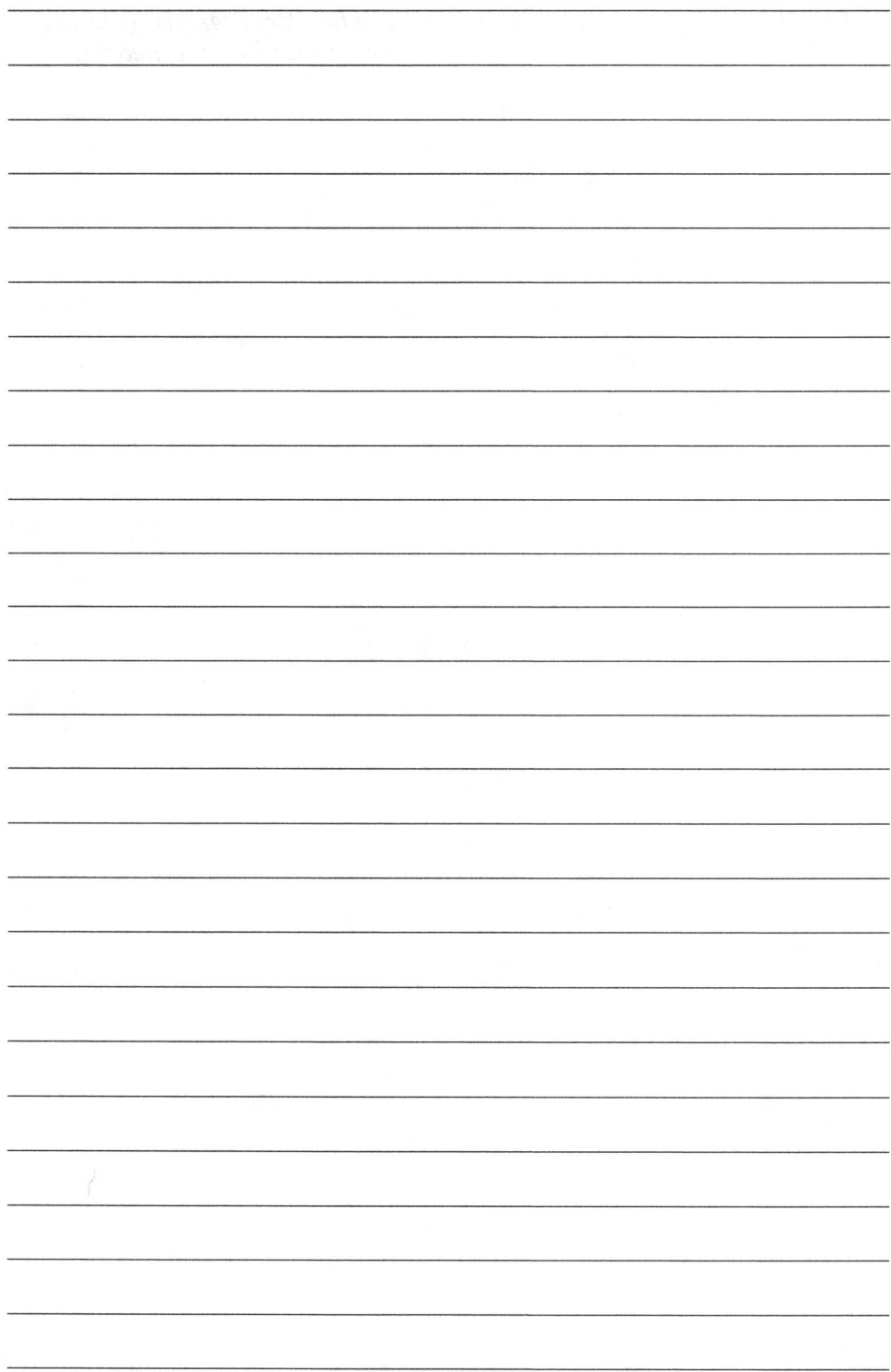

*Water is the most neglected nutrient in your diet,*
*but one of the most vital.*

– Julia Child

_____

_____

_____

_____

_____

_____

_____

_____

_____

_____

_____

_____

_____

_____

_____

_____

_____

_____

_____

_____

_____

_____

_____

_____

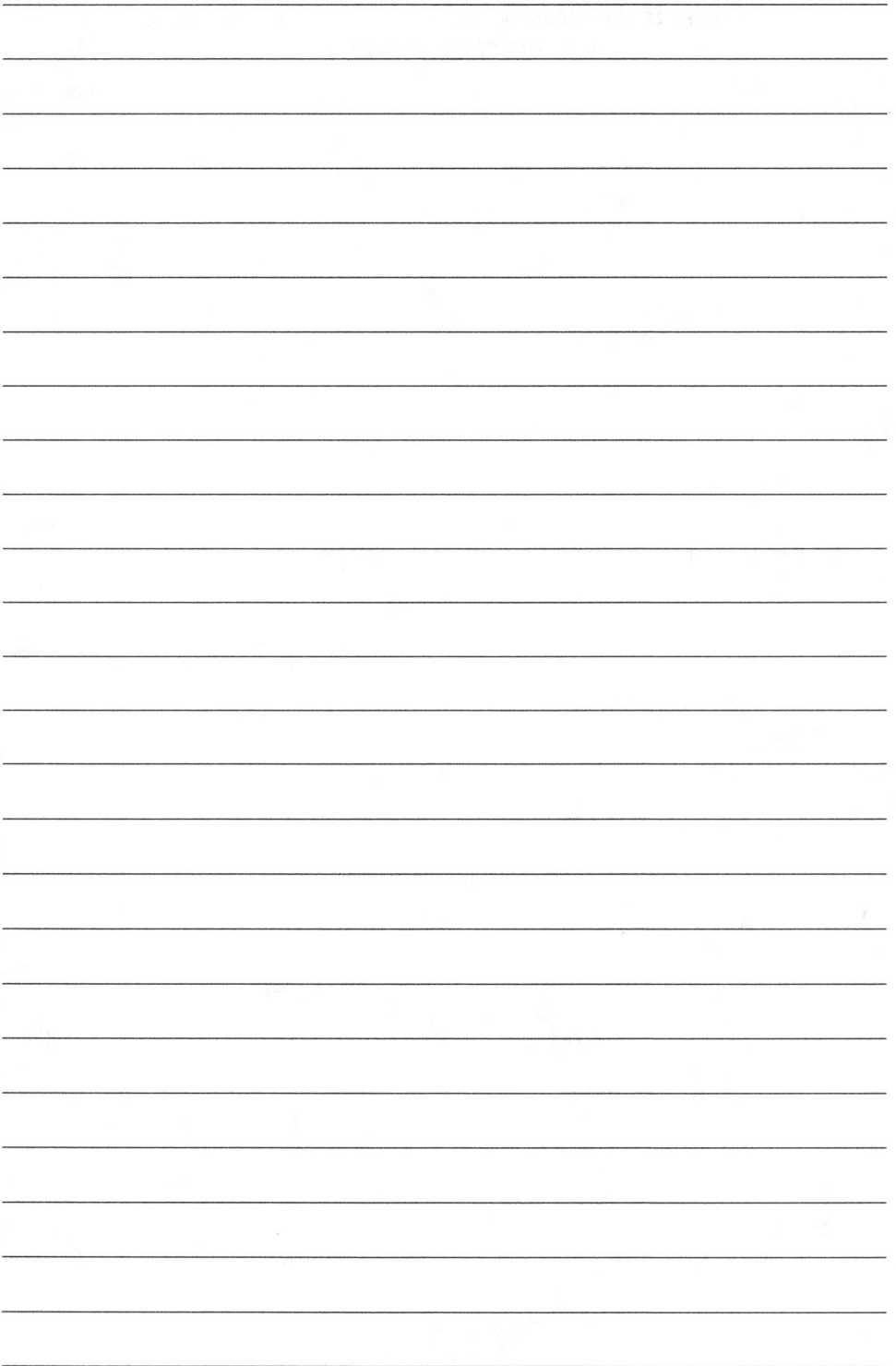

*Let food be thy medicine and medicine be thy food.*

– Hippocrates

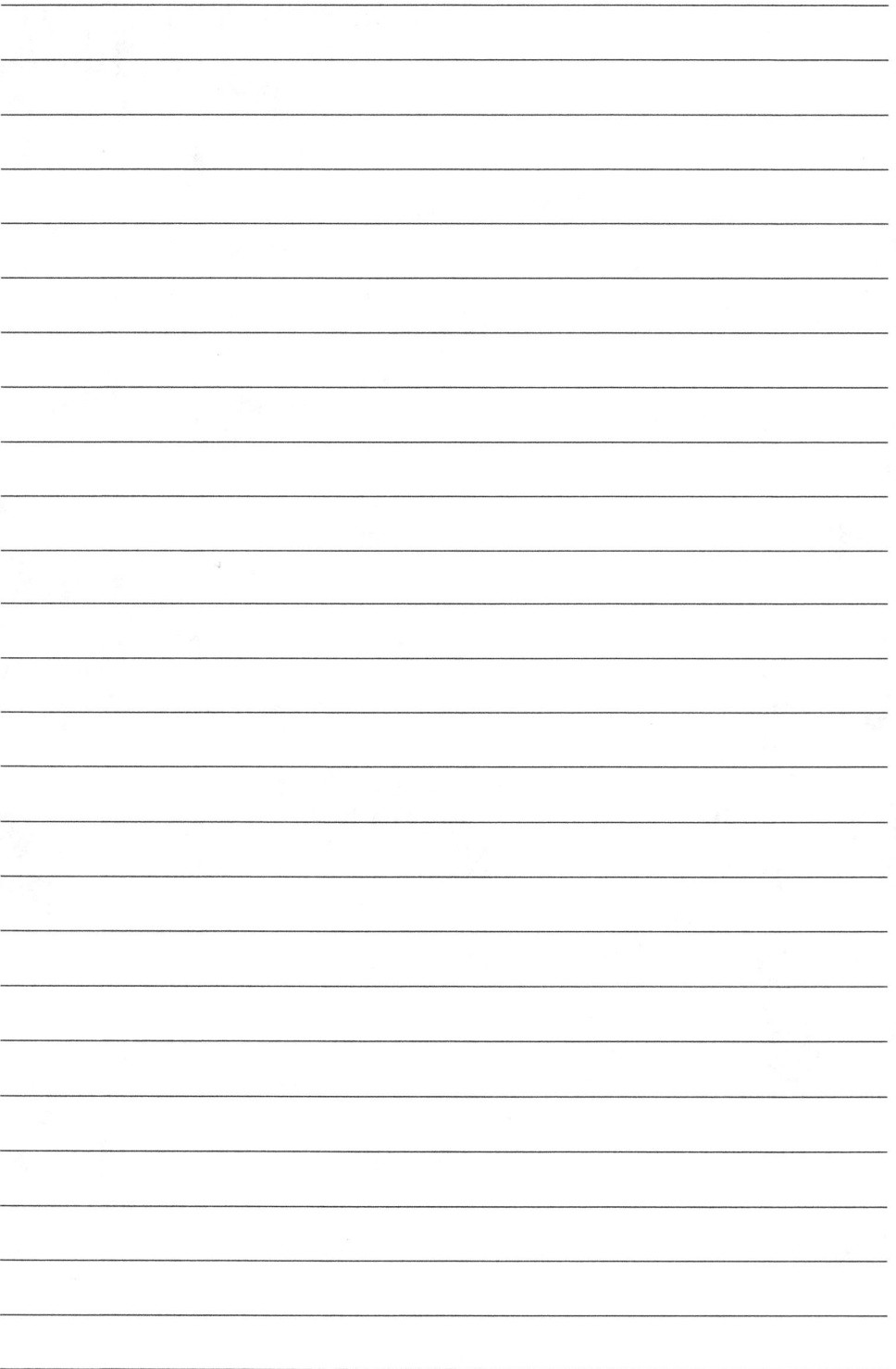

*The food you eat can be either the safest and most powerful form of medicine or the slowest form of poison.*

– Ann Wigmore

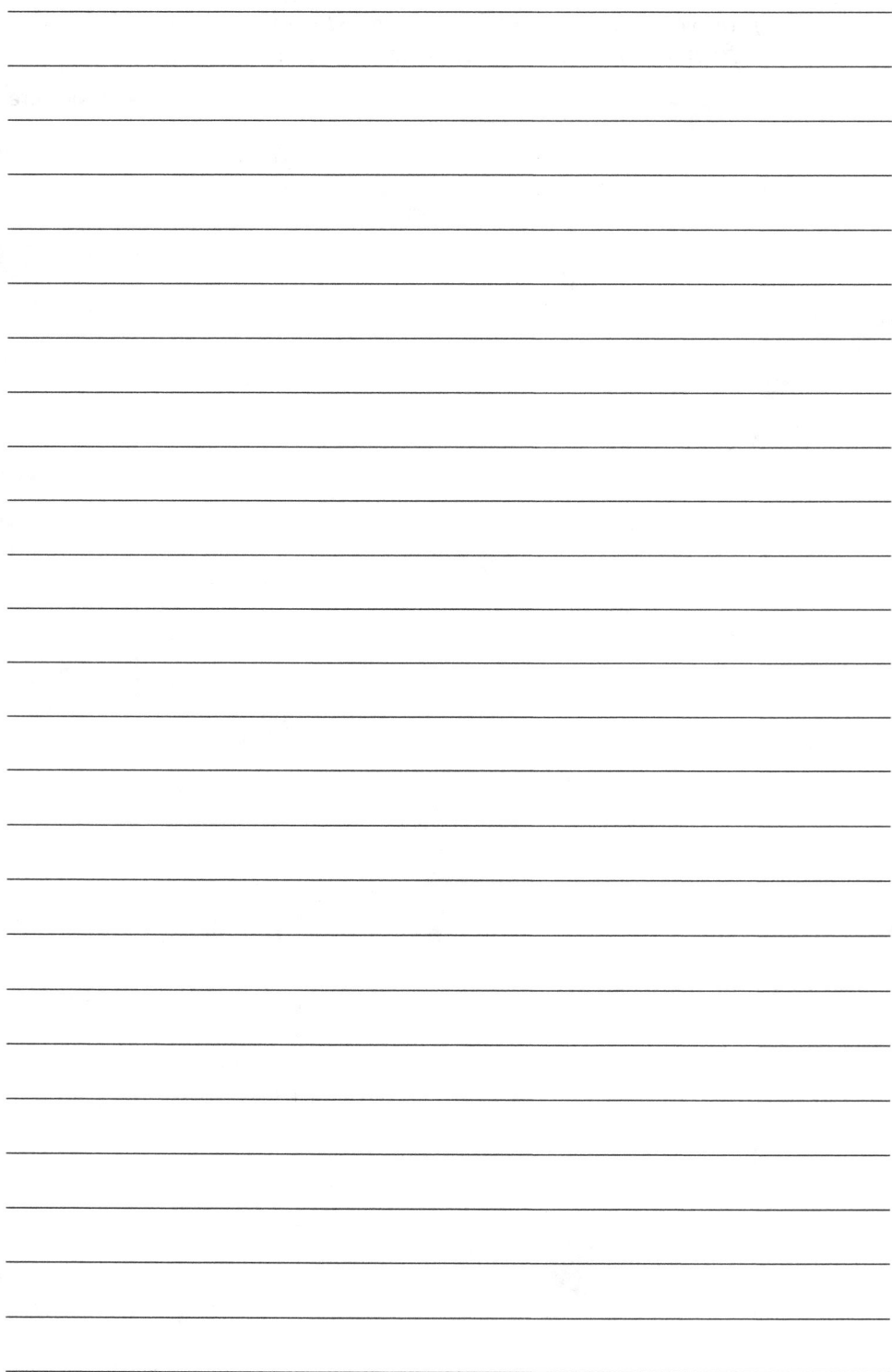

*Exercise is King, nutrition is Queen,*
*put them together and you've got a kingdom.*

– Jack LaLanne

_____

_____

_____

_____

_____

_____

_____

_____

_____

_____

_____

_____

_____

_____

_____

_____

_____

_____

_____

_____

_____

_____

_____

_____

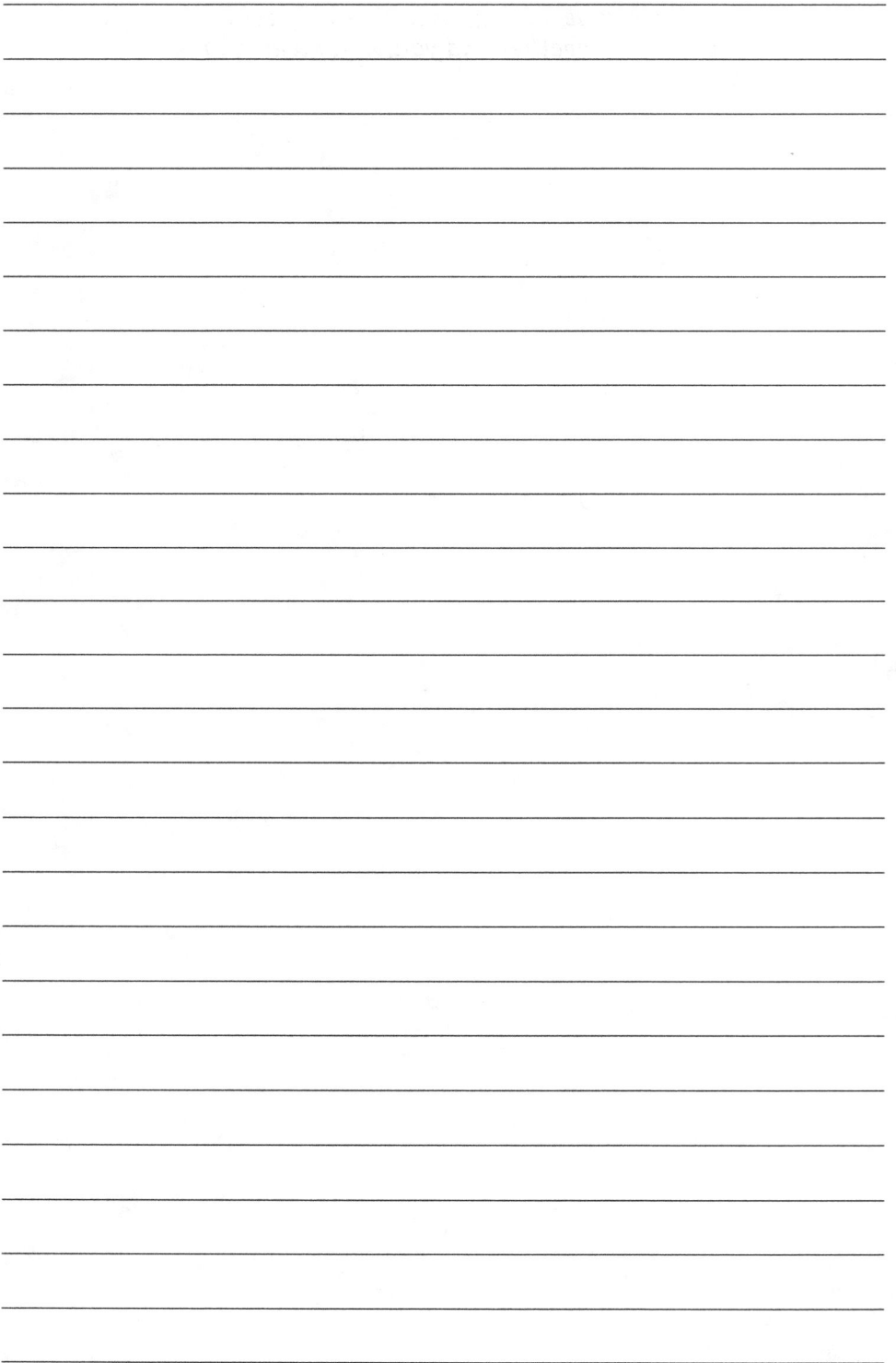

*Obesity is not because it runs in the family,
it's because, no one runs in the family.*

– Anonymous

_____

_____

_____

_____

_____

_____

_____

_____

_____

_____

_____

_____

_____

_____

_____

_____

_____

_____

_____

_____

_____

_____

_____

_____

_____

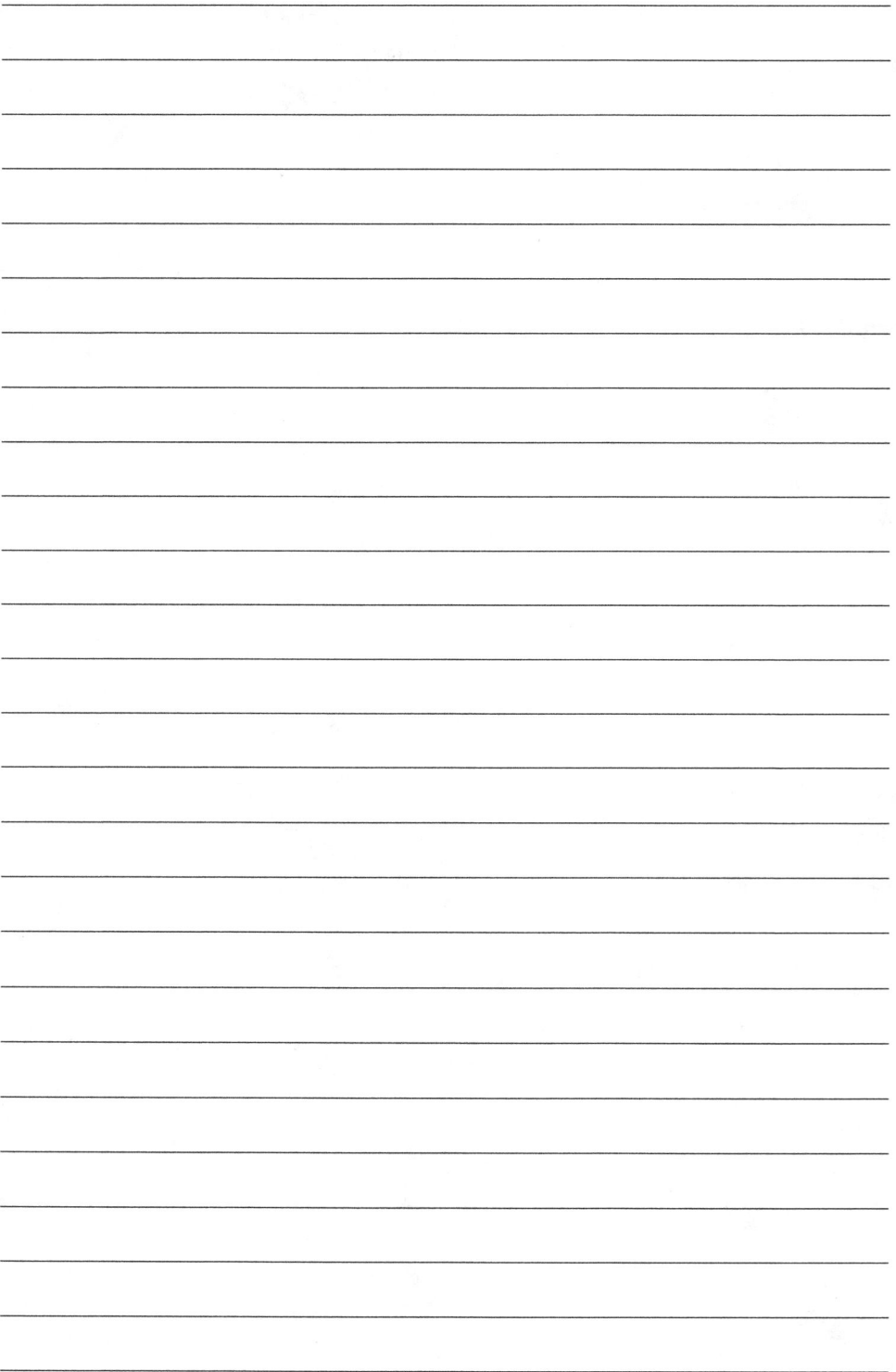

*Tip 16: Become more active by finding activities
you and your family enjoy. Joining a gym is not necessary
as you can go for walks, run, or a bike ride.*

_____

_____

_____

_____

_____

_____

_____

_____

_____

_____

_____

_____

_____

_____

_____

_____

_____

_____

_____

_____

_____

_____

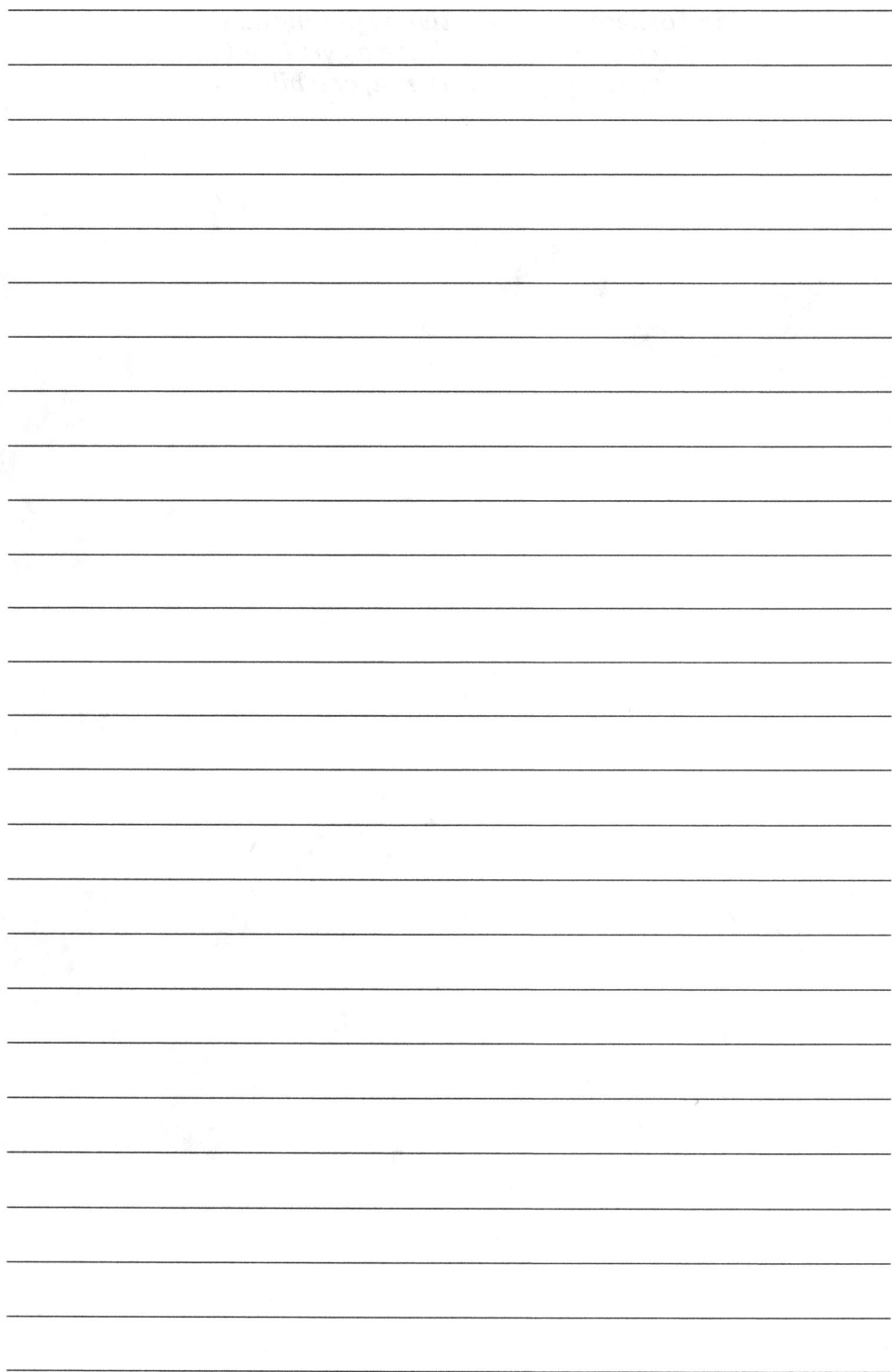

*Exercise is so amazing from the inside out.*
*I feel so alive and have so much energy.*

– Vanessa Hudgens

_____

_____

_____

_____

_____

_____

_____

_____

_____

_____

_____

_____

_____

_____

_____

_____

_____

_____

_____

_____

_____

_____

_____

_____

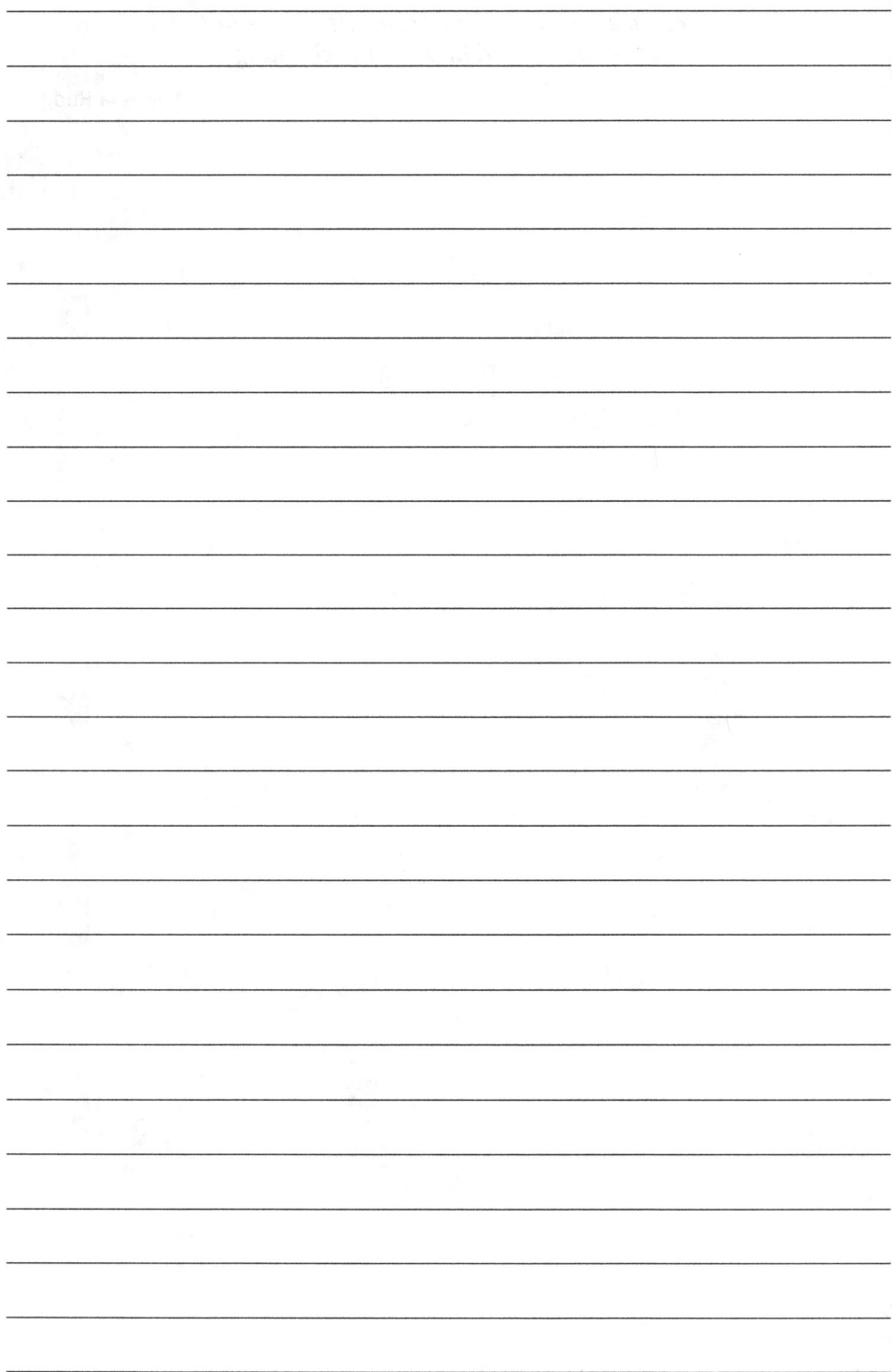

*It is better to take many small steps in the right direction than to make a great leap forward only to stumble backward.*

– Old Chinese Proverb

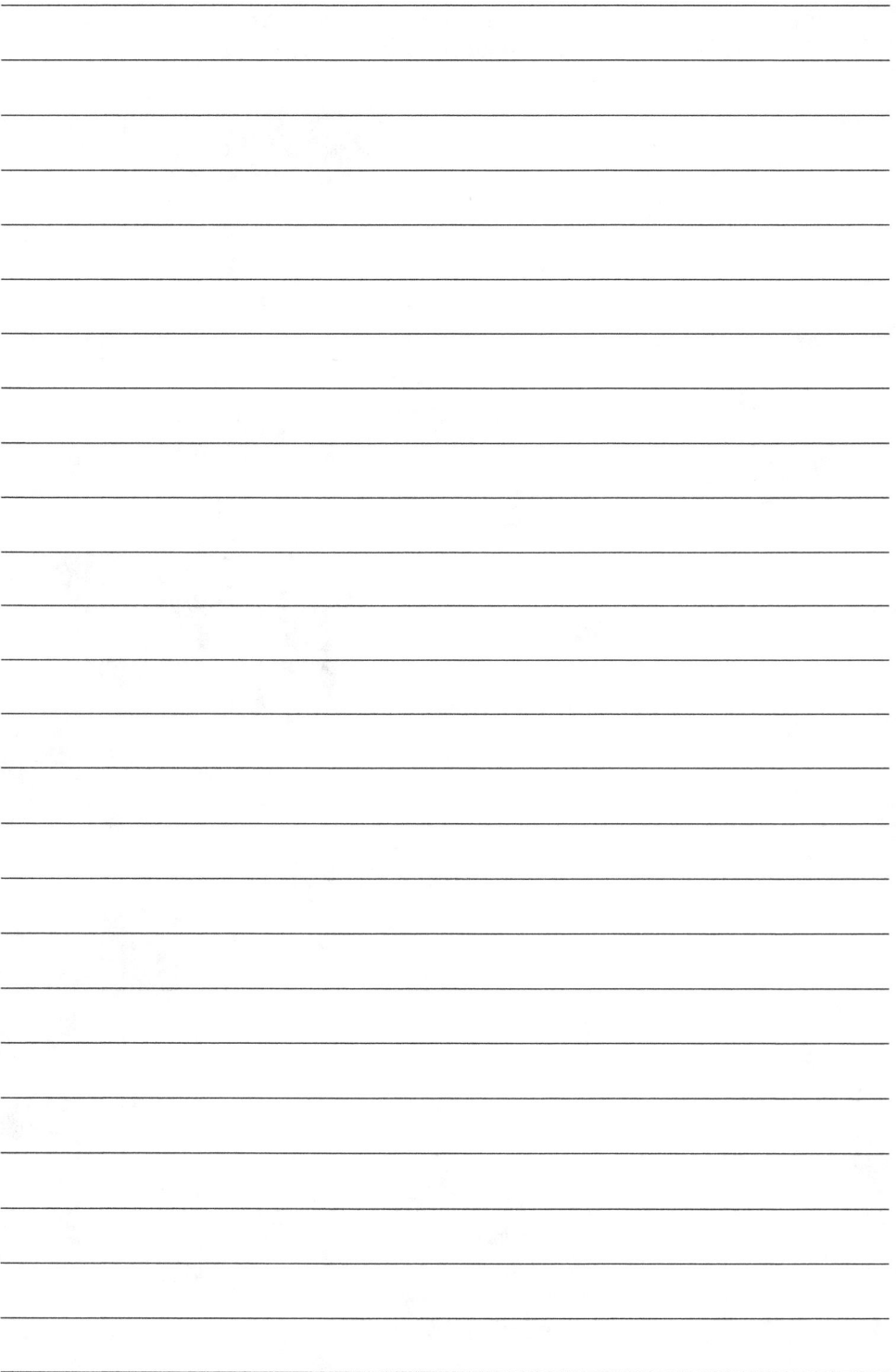

*Great things are not done by impulse,*
*but by a series of small things brought together.*

– Vincent Van Gogh

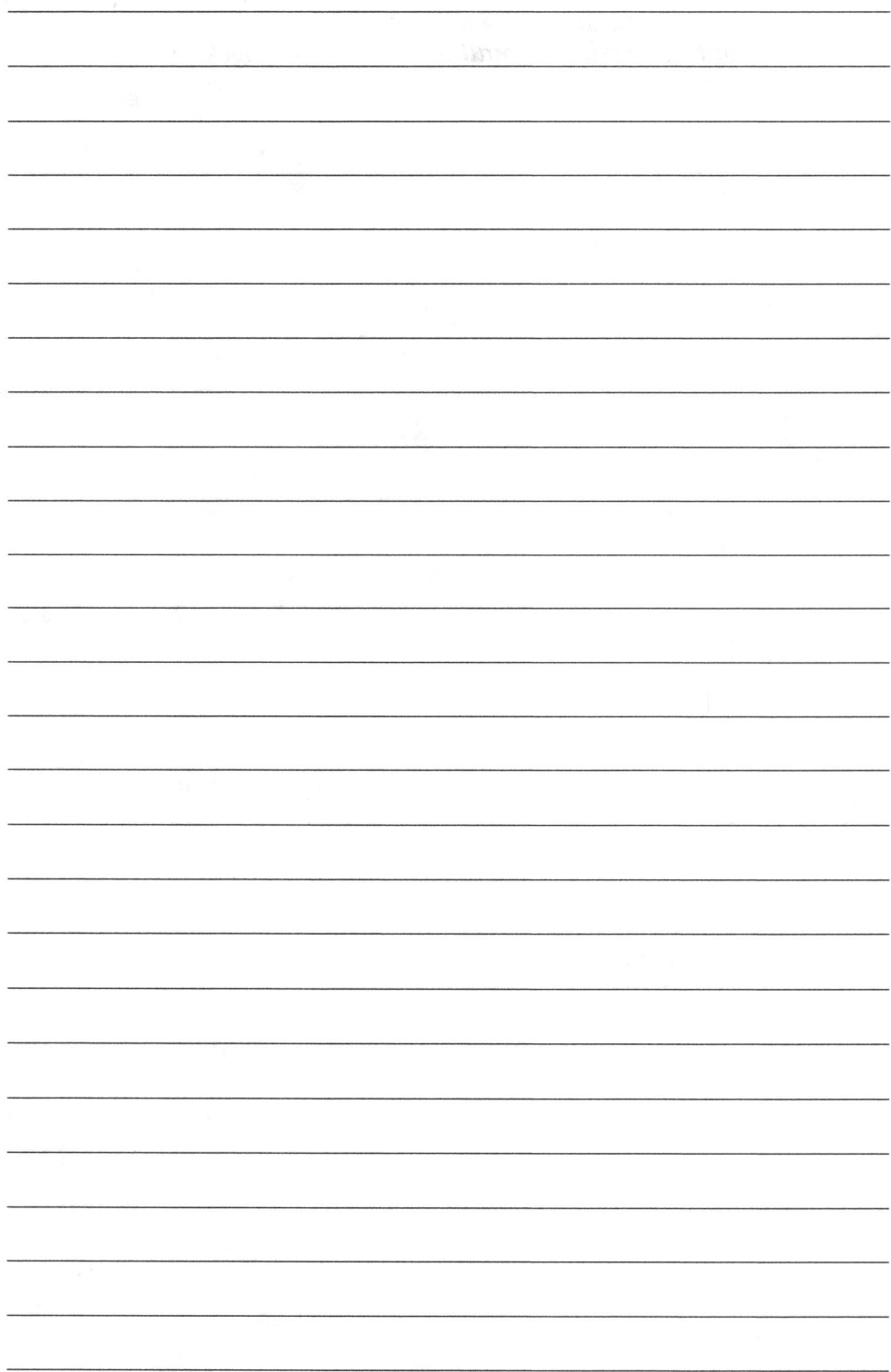

*You will never change your life until you change something you do daily.*

– Mike Murdock

_____

_____

_____

_____

_____

_____

_____

_____

_____

_____

_____

_____

_____

_____

_____

_____

_____

_____

_____

_____

_____

_____

_____

_____

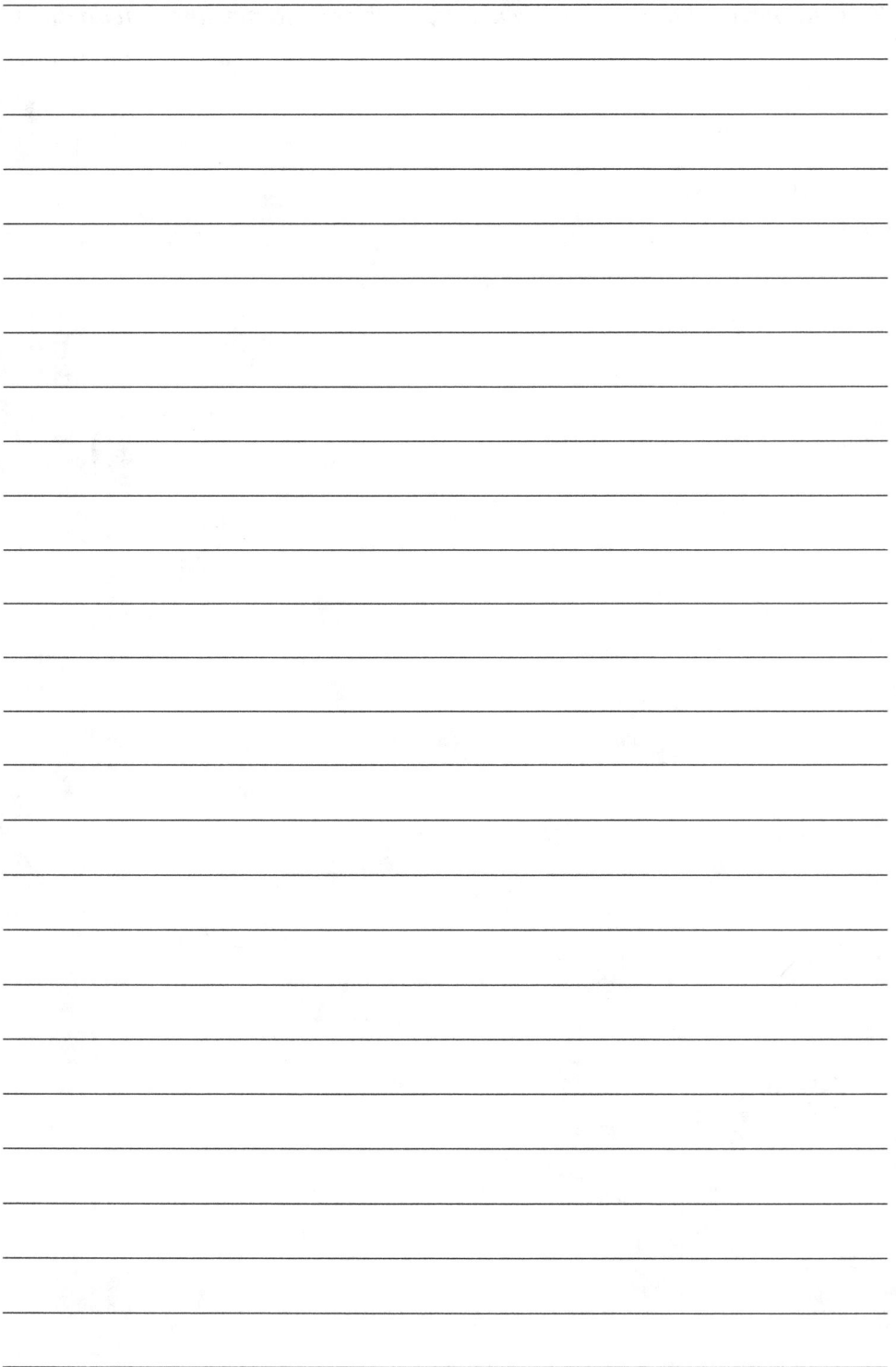

*Habit is habit and not to be flung out of the window by any man,*
*but coaxed downstairs a step at a time.*

– Mark Twain

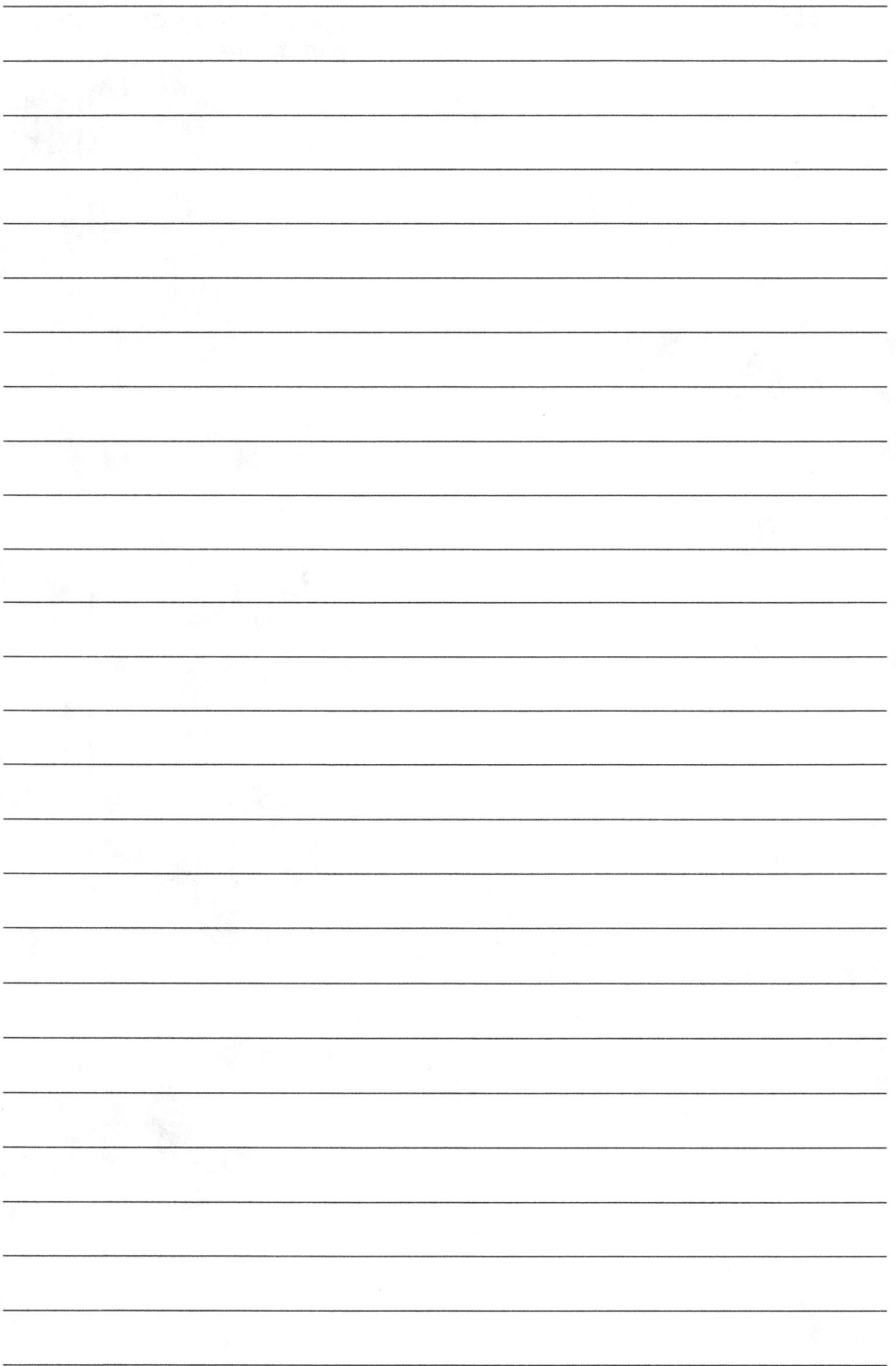

*Tip 17: Avoid process foods. They tend to be high in sugar,
salt, and fats, and contain little nutrients.*

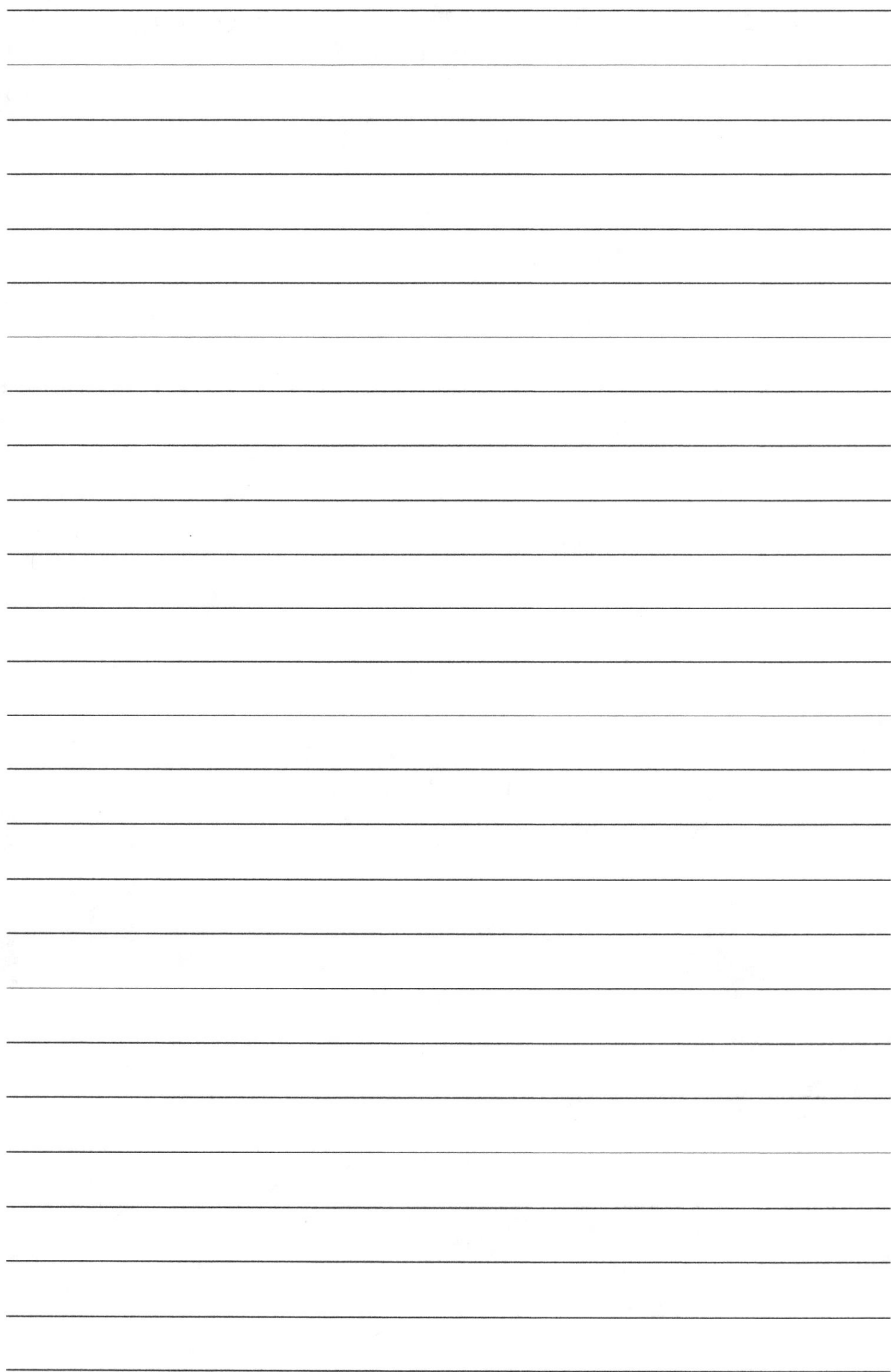

*Processed foods not only extend the shelf life,*
*but they extend the waistline as well.*

– Karen Sessions

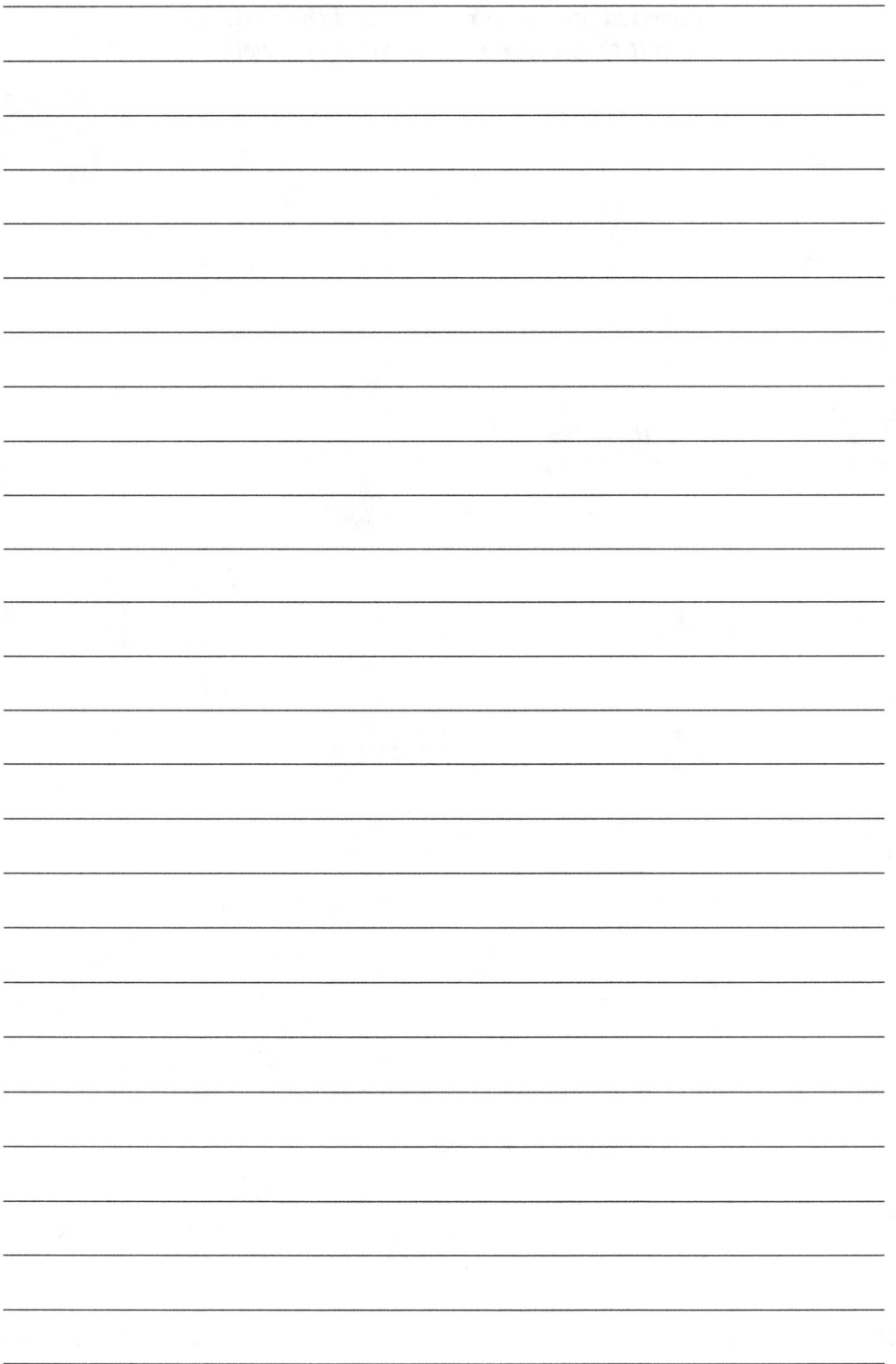

*Can it be a mistake that 'STRESSED' is 'DESSERTS' spelled backwards?*

– Unknown

_____

_____

_____

_____

_____

_____

_____

_____

_____

_____

_____

_____

_____

_____

_____

_____

_____

_____

_____

_____

_____

_____

_____

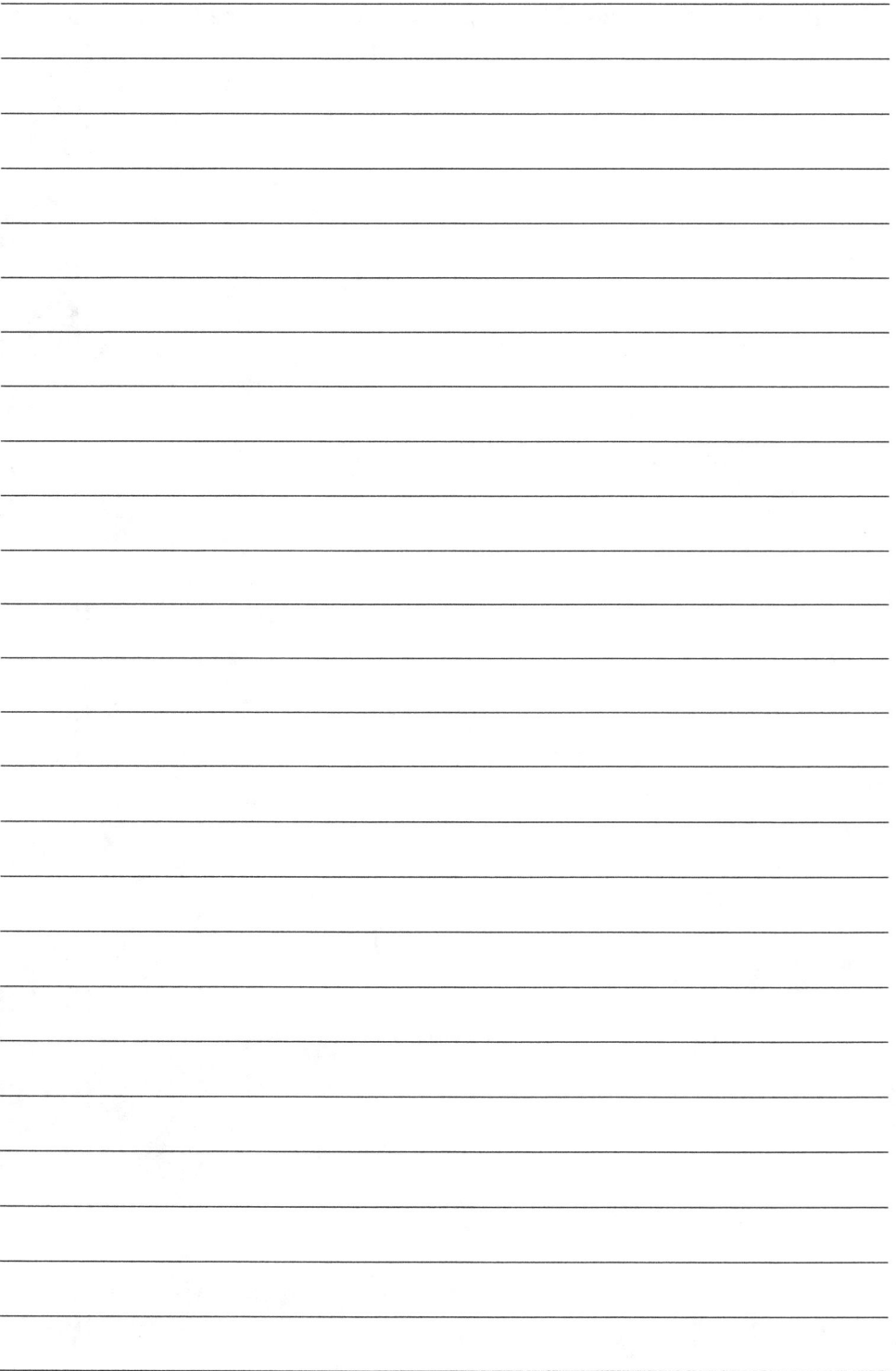

*Don't eat anything your great-great grandmother*
*wouldn't recognize as food.*

– Michael Pollan

_____

_____

_____

_____

_____

_____

_____

_____

_____

_____

_____

_____

_____

_____

_____

_____

_____

_____

_____

_____

_____

_____

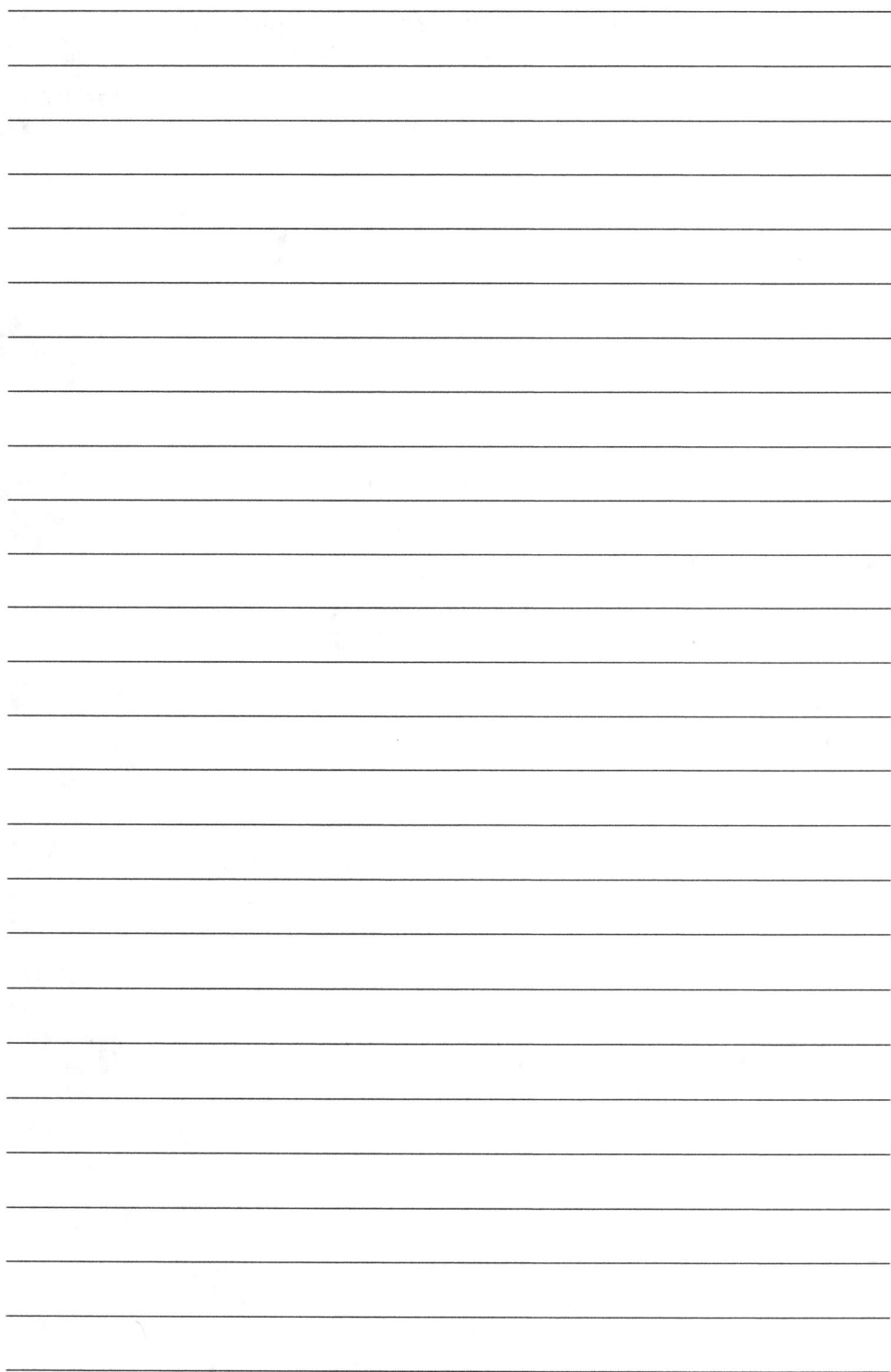

*First thing every morning before you arise, say out loud,*
*'I believe', three times.*

– Norman Vincent Peal

_____

_____

_____

_____

_____

_____

_____

_____

_____

_____

_____

_____

_____

_____

_____

_____

_____

_____

_____

_____

_____

_____

_____

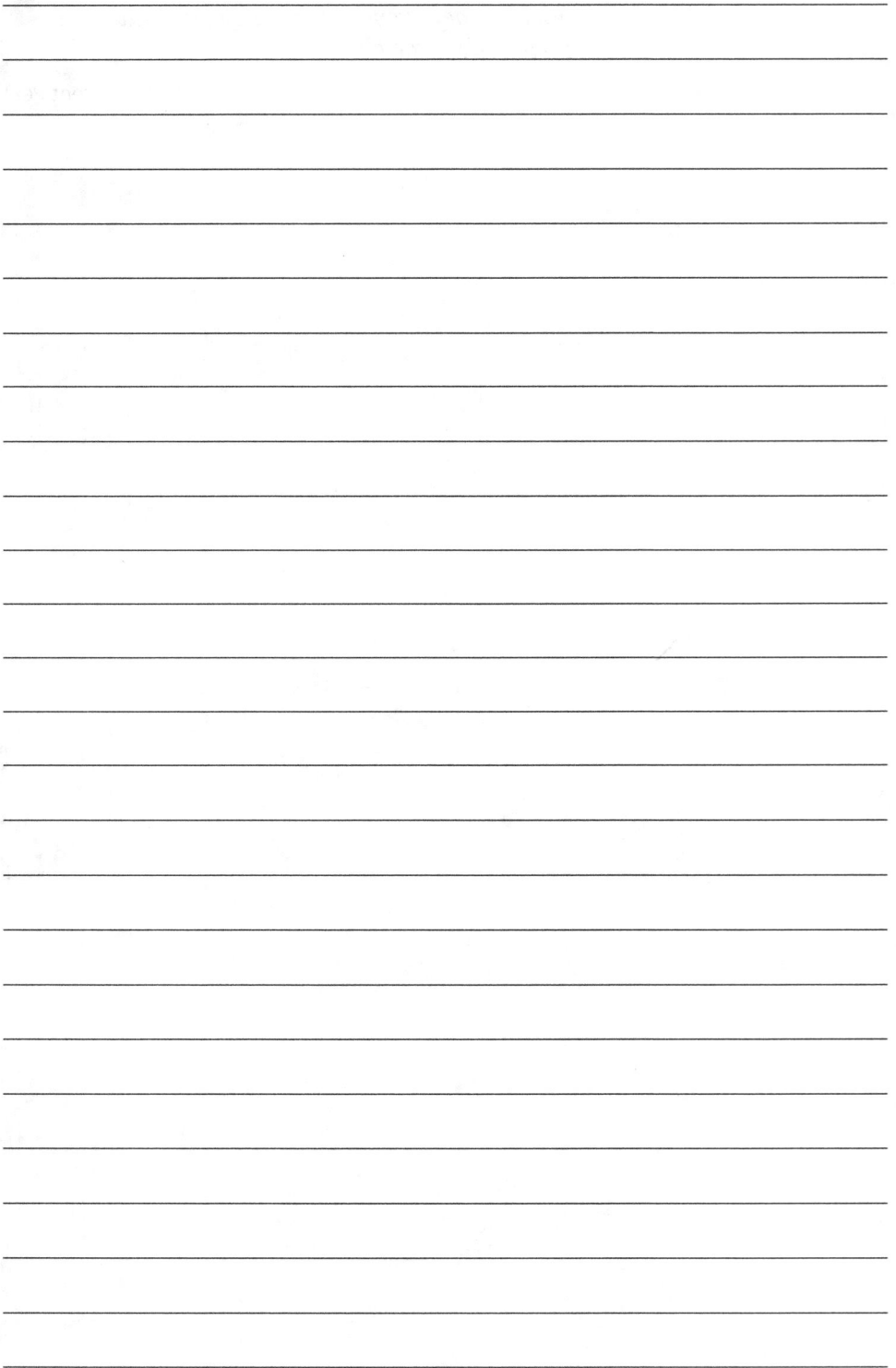

*A diet is a plan, generally hopeless, for reducing your weight, which tests your will power but does little for your waistline.*

– Herbert B. Prochnow

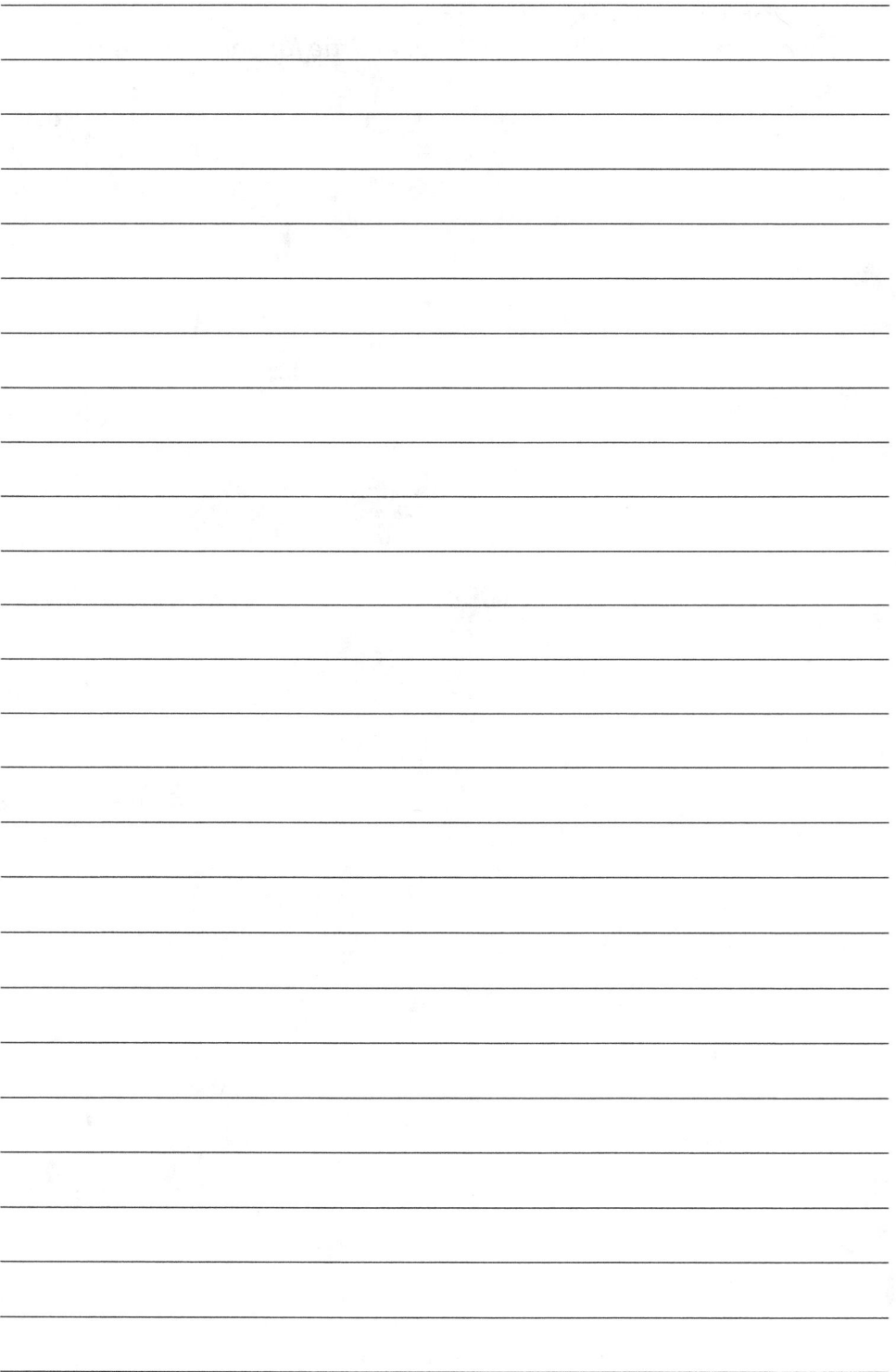

*Tip 18: Consider including intermittent fasting (IF) in your lifestyle. IF includes periods of eating and periods of fasting. There are a variety of methods but they are generally associated with reduced calorie intake.*

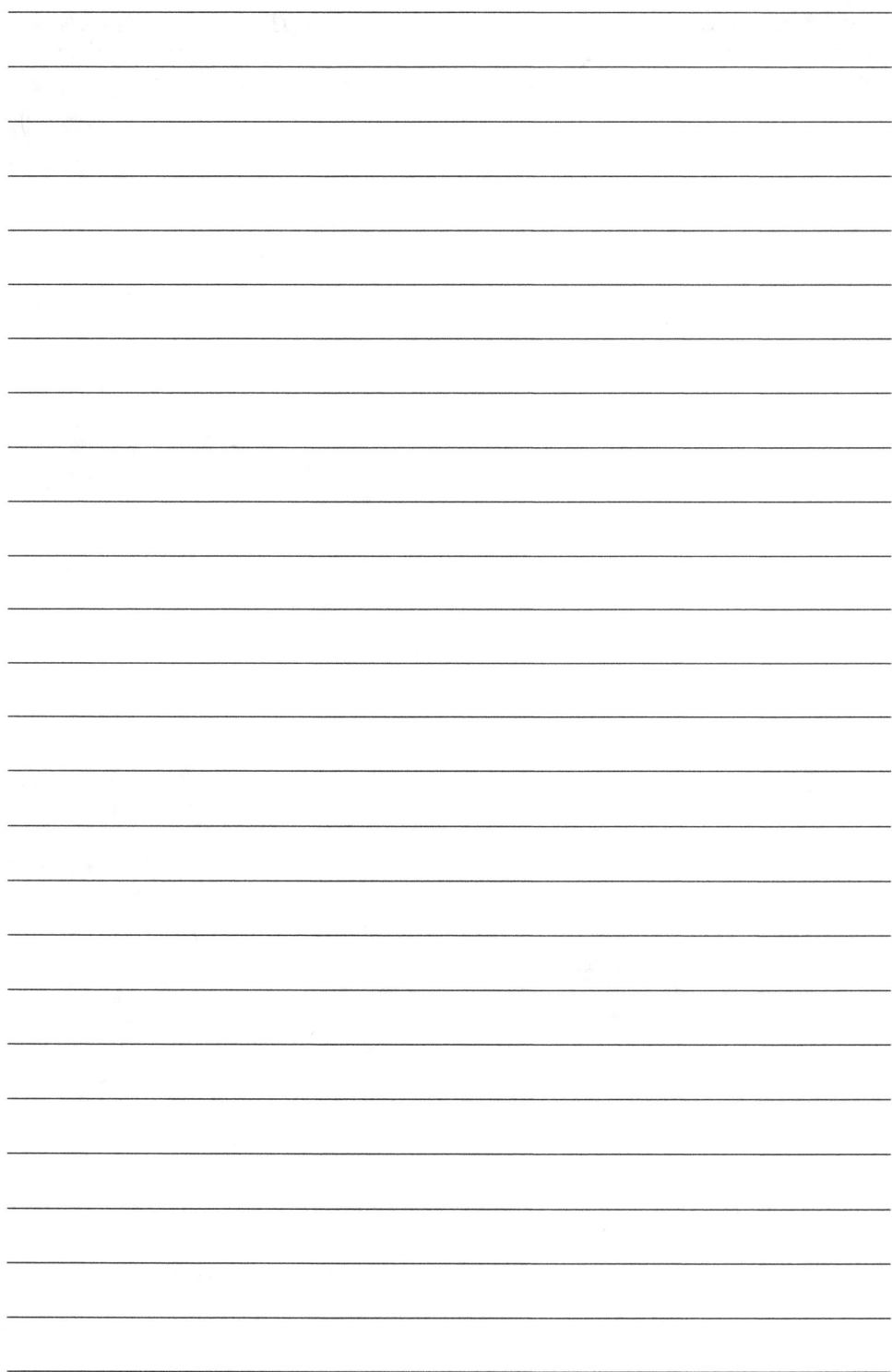

*Health is a state of complete physical, mental and social well-being,*
*and not merely the absence of disease or infirmity.*

– World Health Organization

_____

_____

_____

_____

_____

_____

_____

_____

_____

_____

_____

_____

_____

_____

_____

_____

_____

_____

_____

_____

_____

_____

_____

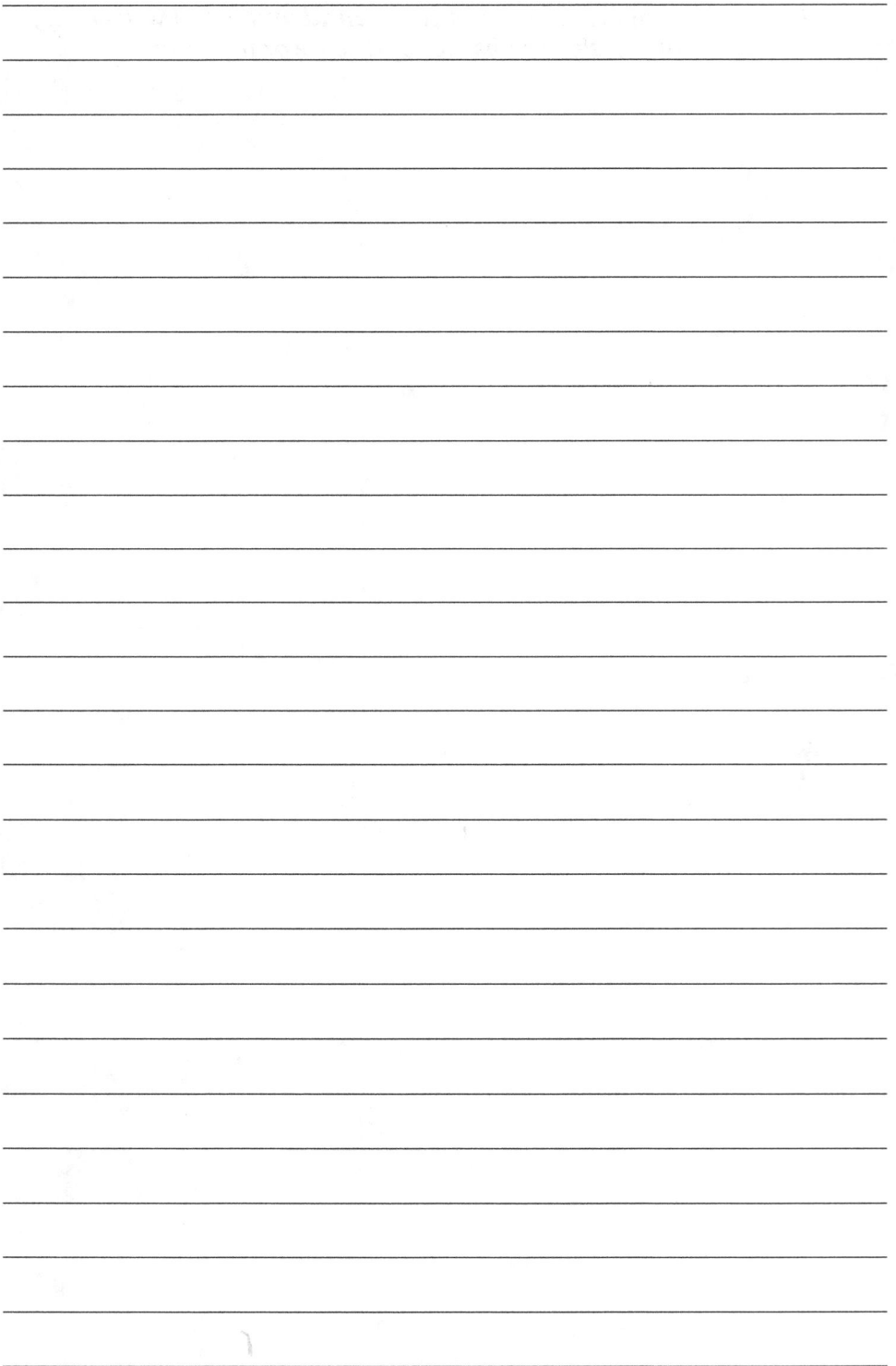

*If food is your best friend, it's also your worst enemy.*

– Edward "Grandpa" Jones

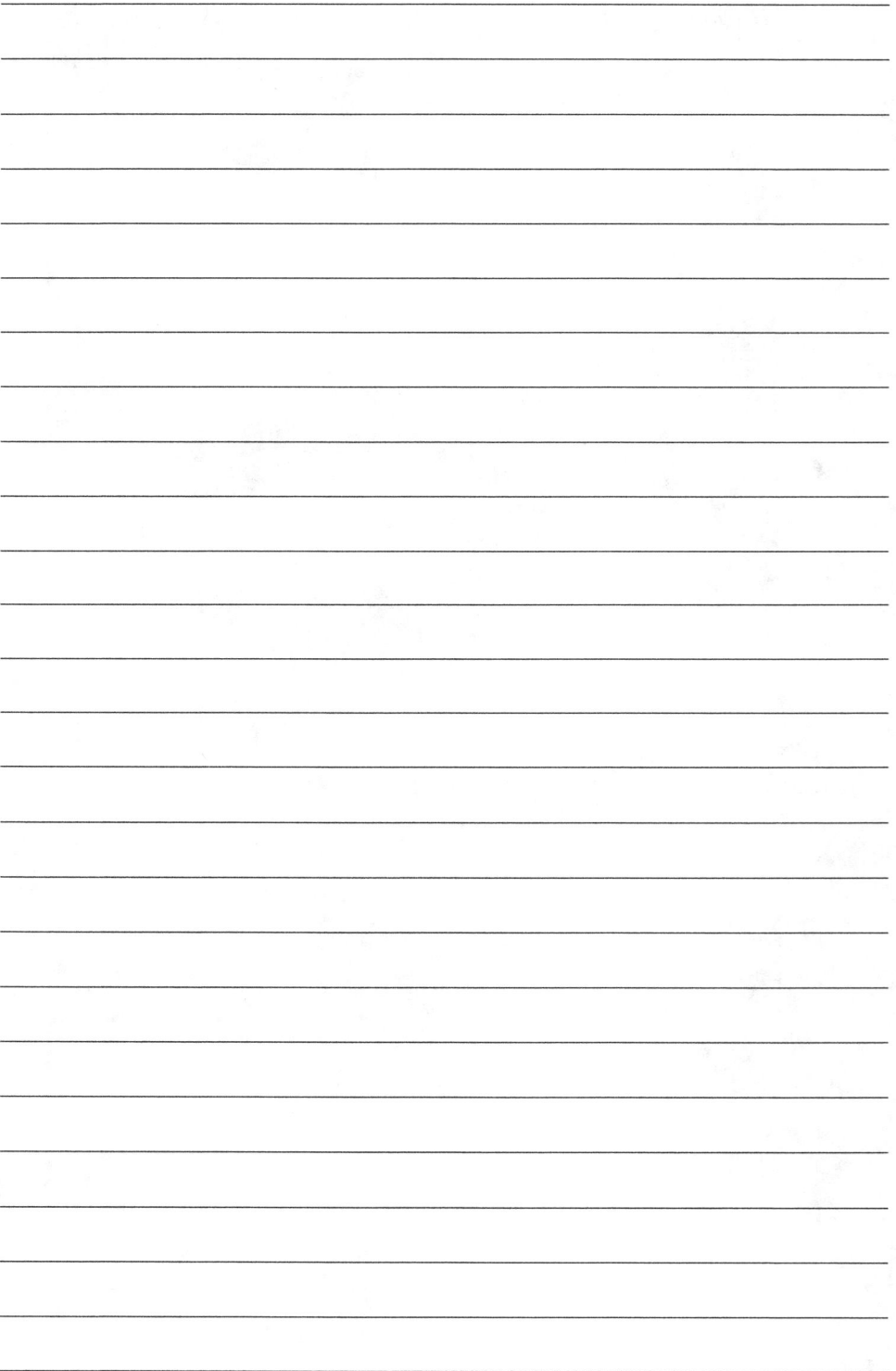

*Tip 19: Add spice to your food. Chili peppers and jalapenos contain a compound called capsaicin, which may boost metabolism and increase the burning of fat.*

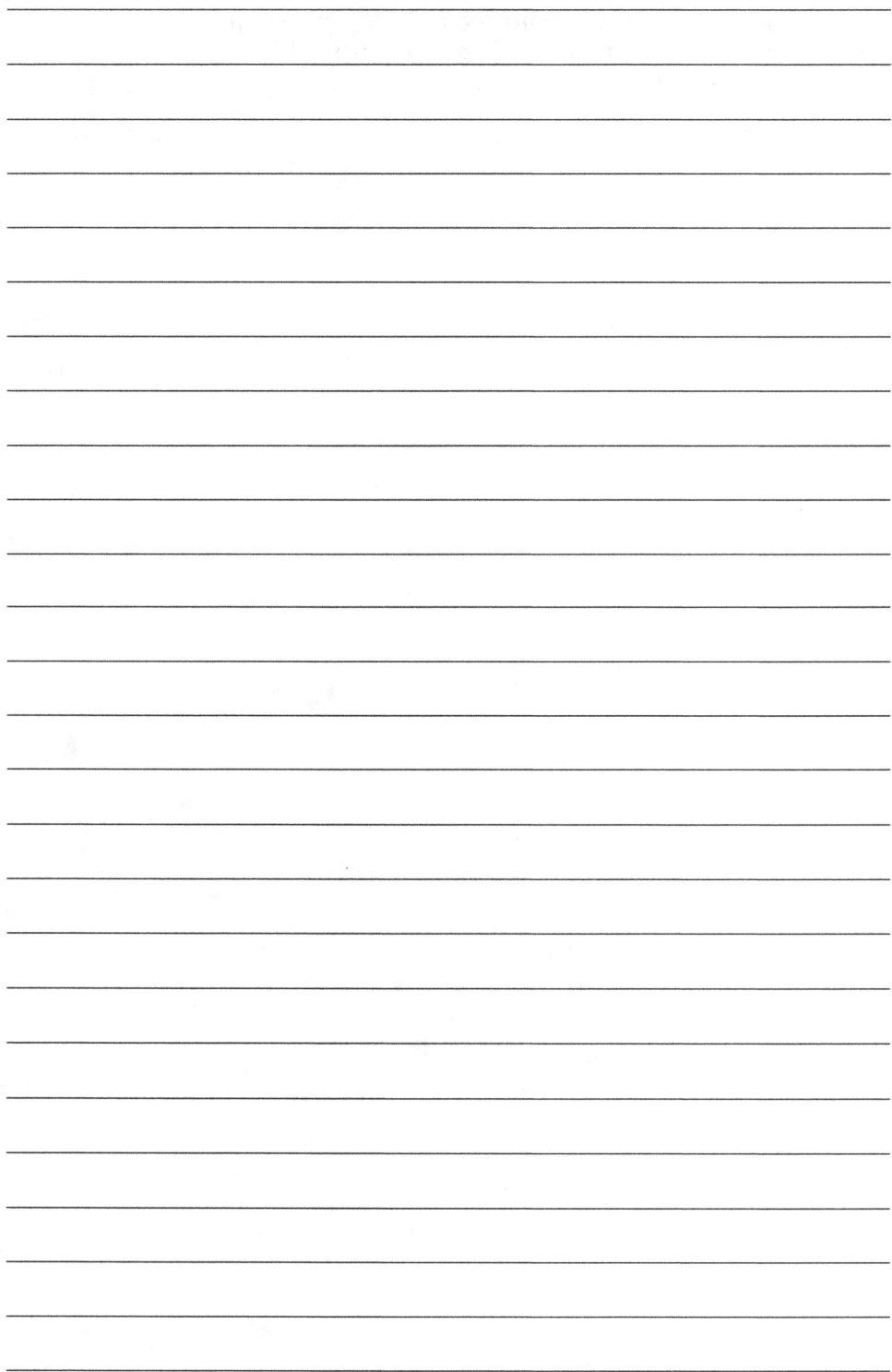

*A man too busy to take care of his health is like*
*a mechanic too busy to take care of his tools.*

– Spanish Proverb

_____

_____

_____

_____

_____

_____

_____

_____

_____

_____

_____

_____

_____

_____

_____

_____

_____

_____

_____

_____

_____

_____

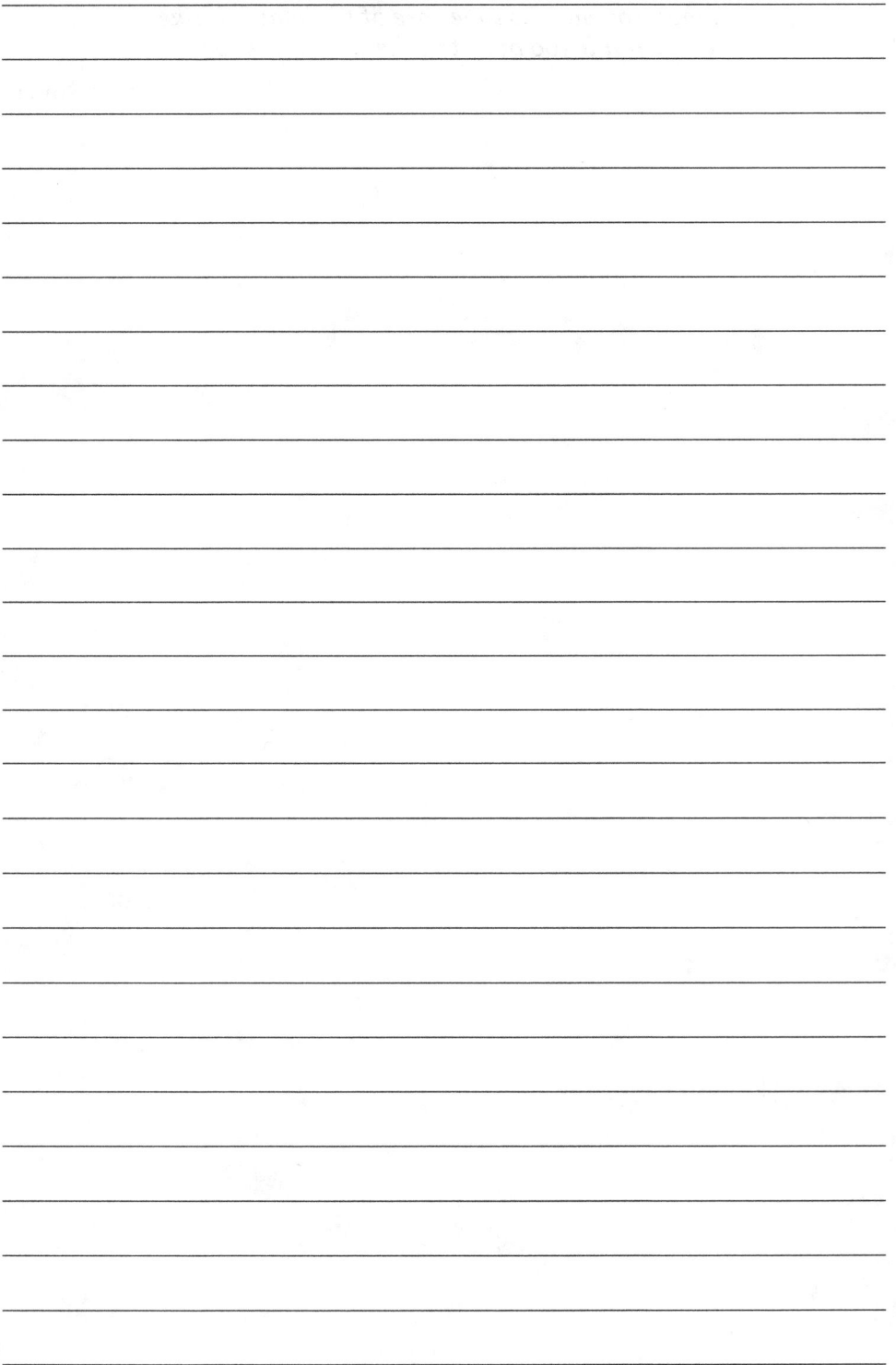

*Put all excuses aside and remember this: YOU are capable.*

– Zig Ziglar

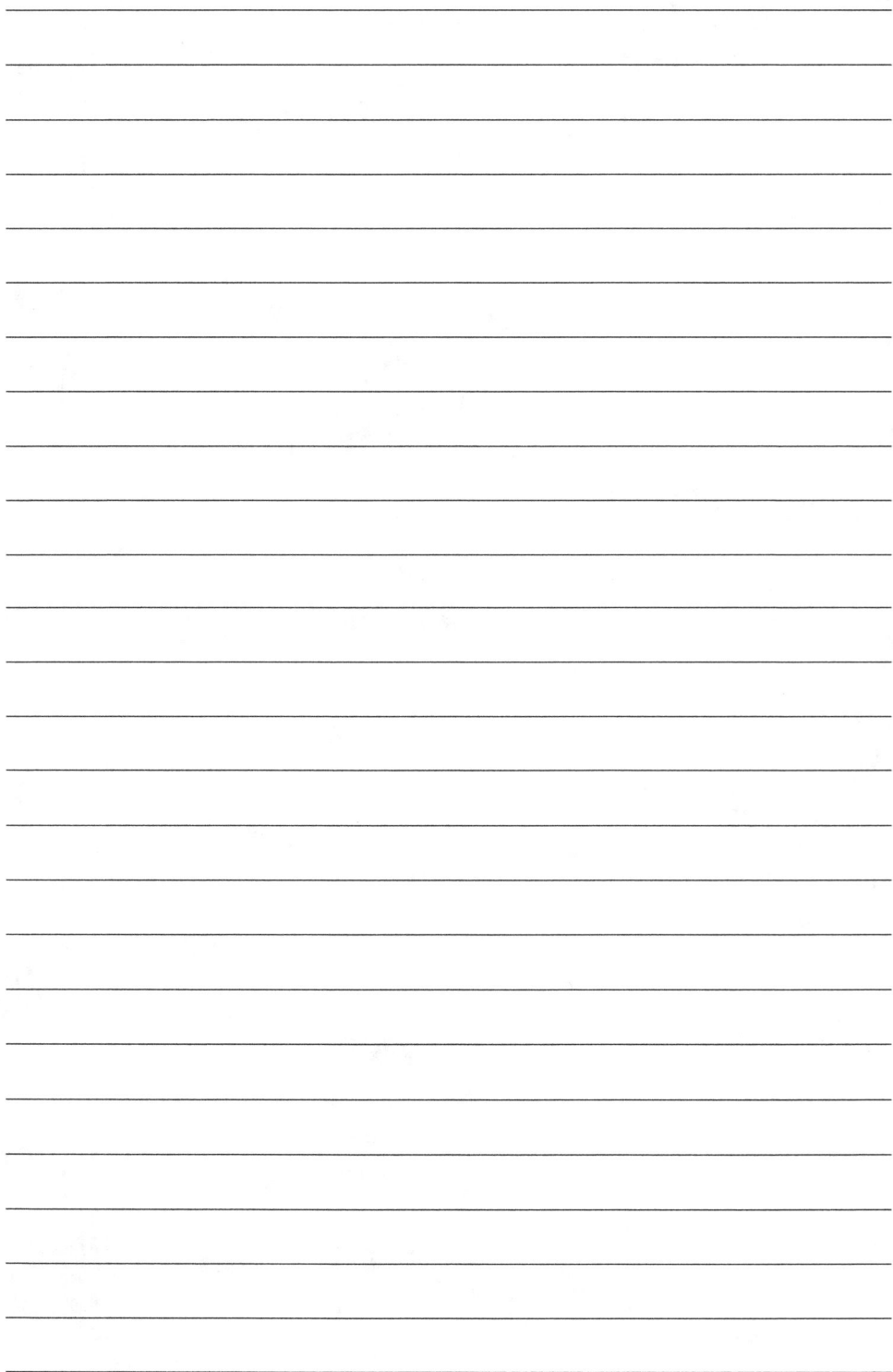

*Look within!... The secret is inside you.*

– Hui-neng

_____

_____

_____

_____

_____

_____

_____

_____

_____

_____

_____

_____

_____

_____

_____

_____

_____

_____

_____

_____

_____

_____

_____

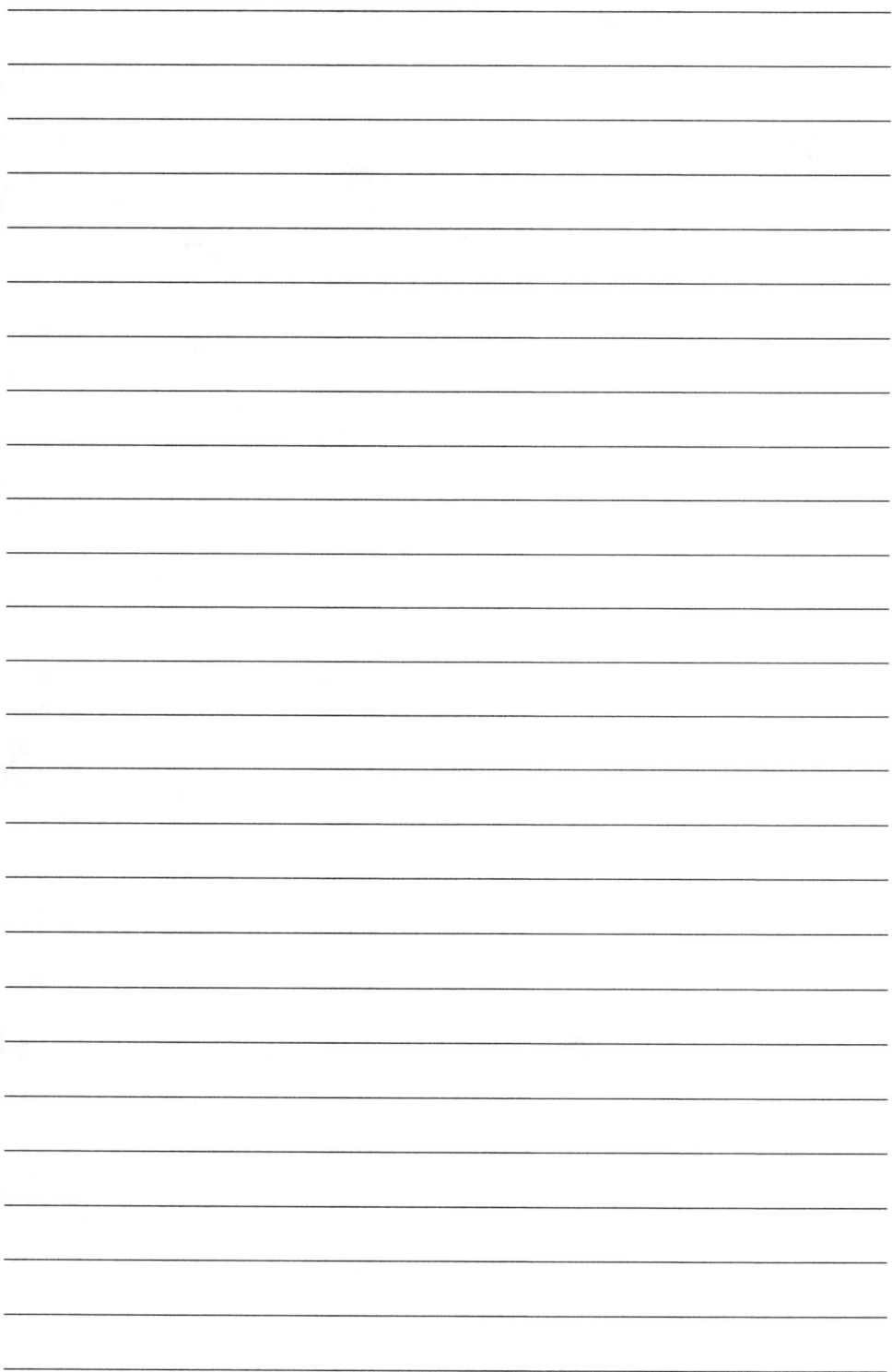

*Tip 20: Practice good sleep hygiene. Studies have shown that sleep-deprived people are up to 55% more likely to become obese, compared to those who get enough sleep.*

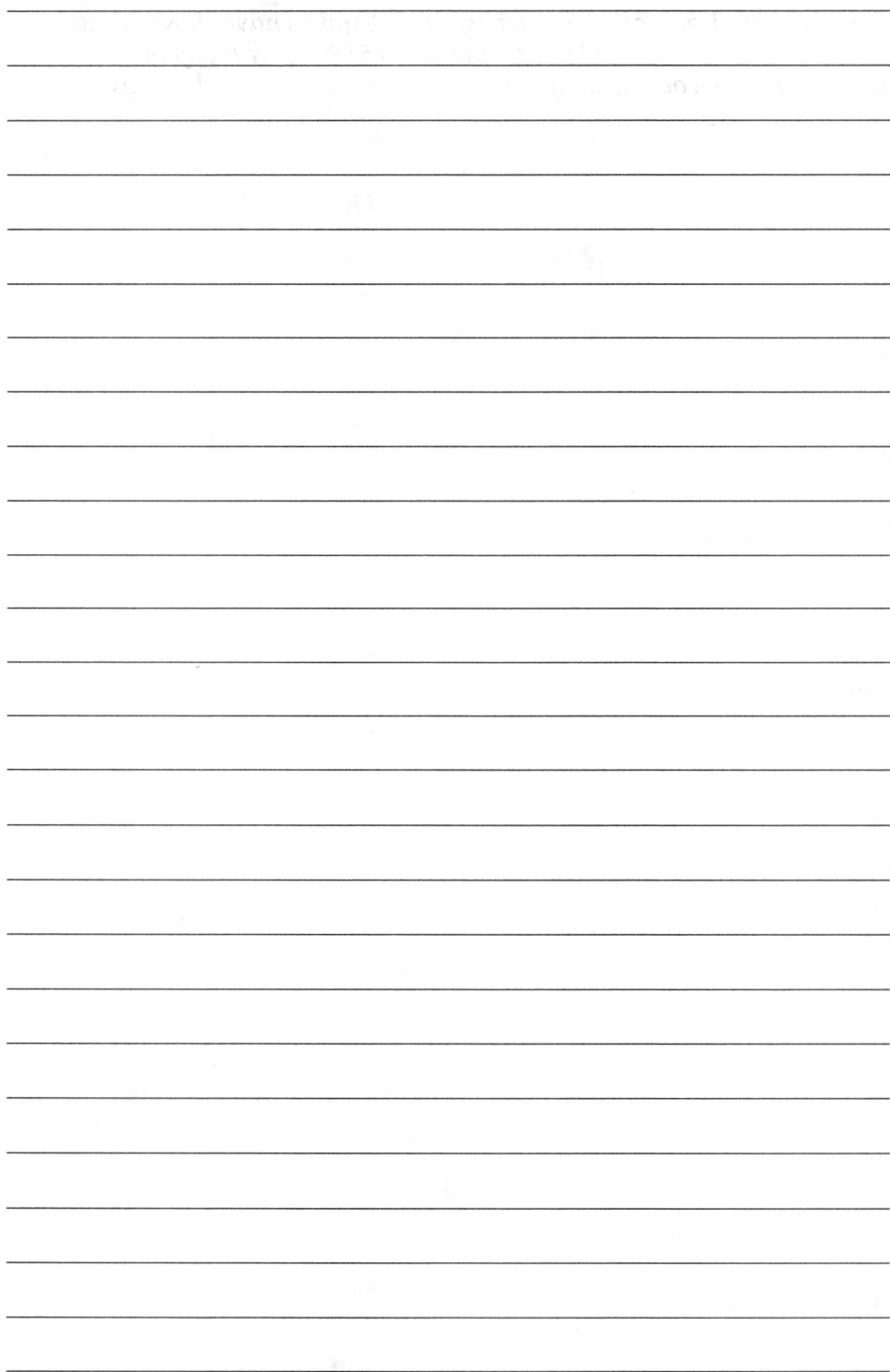

*You must take personal responsibility. You cannot change the circumstances, the seasons, or the wind, but you can change yourself.*

– Jim Rohn

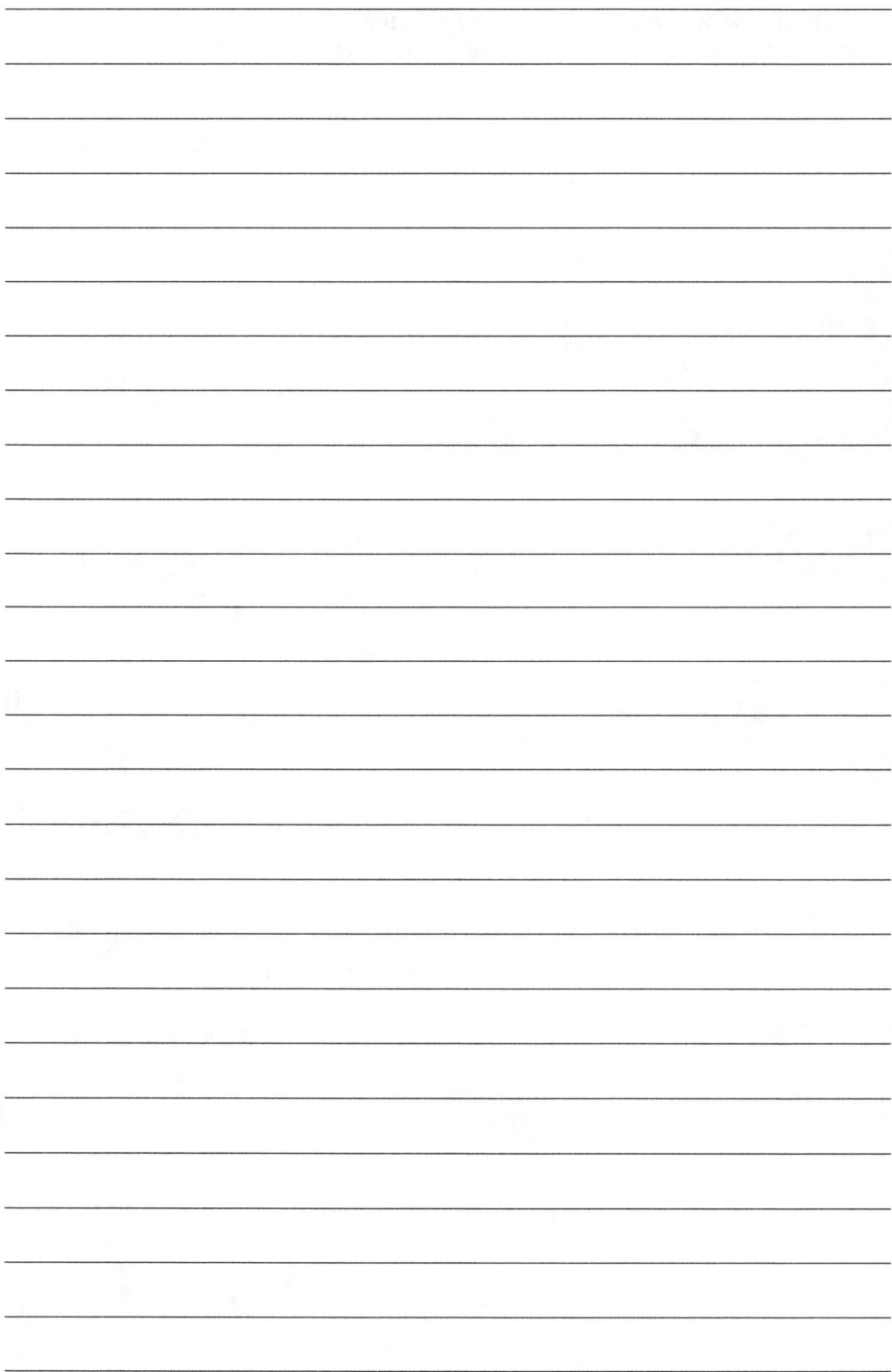

*There are two primary choices in life: to accept conditions as they exist, or accept the responsibility for changing them.*

– Dr. Denis Waitley

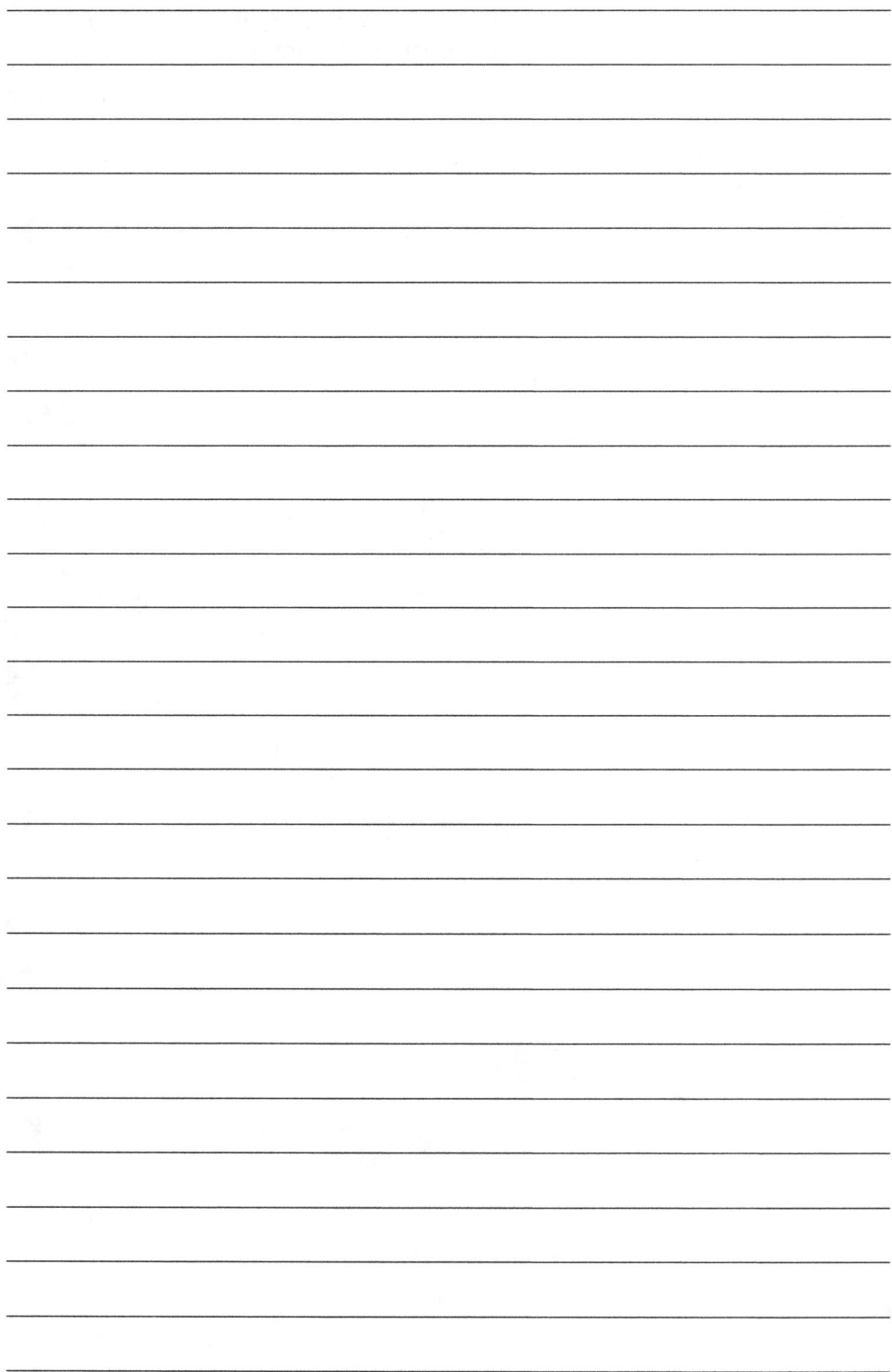

*If you're trying to achieve, there will be roadblocks. I've had them; everybody has had them. But obstacles don't have to stop you. If you run into a wall, don't turn around and give up. Figure out how to climb it, go through it, or work around it.*

– Michael Jordan

*If you don't do what's best for your body,
you're the one who comes up on the short end.*

– Julius Erving

_____

_____

_____

_____

_____

_____

_____

_____

_____

_____

_____

_____

_____

_____

_____

_____

_____

_____

_____

_____

_____

_____

_____

_____

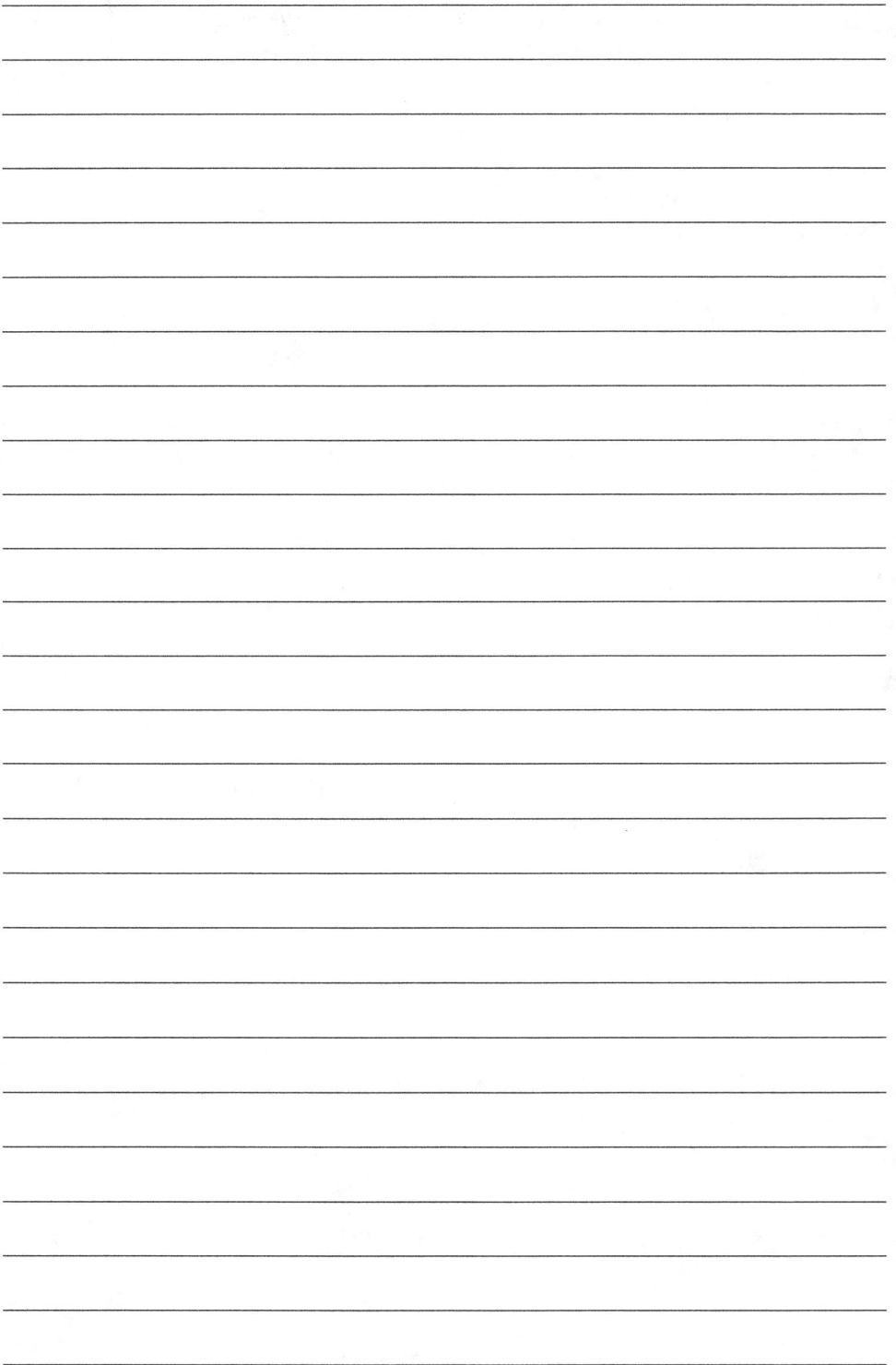

*Junk food satisfies you for a minute, being fit satisfies you for life.*

– Unknown

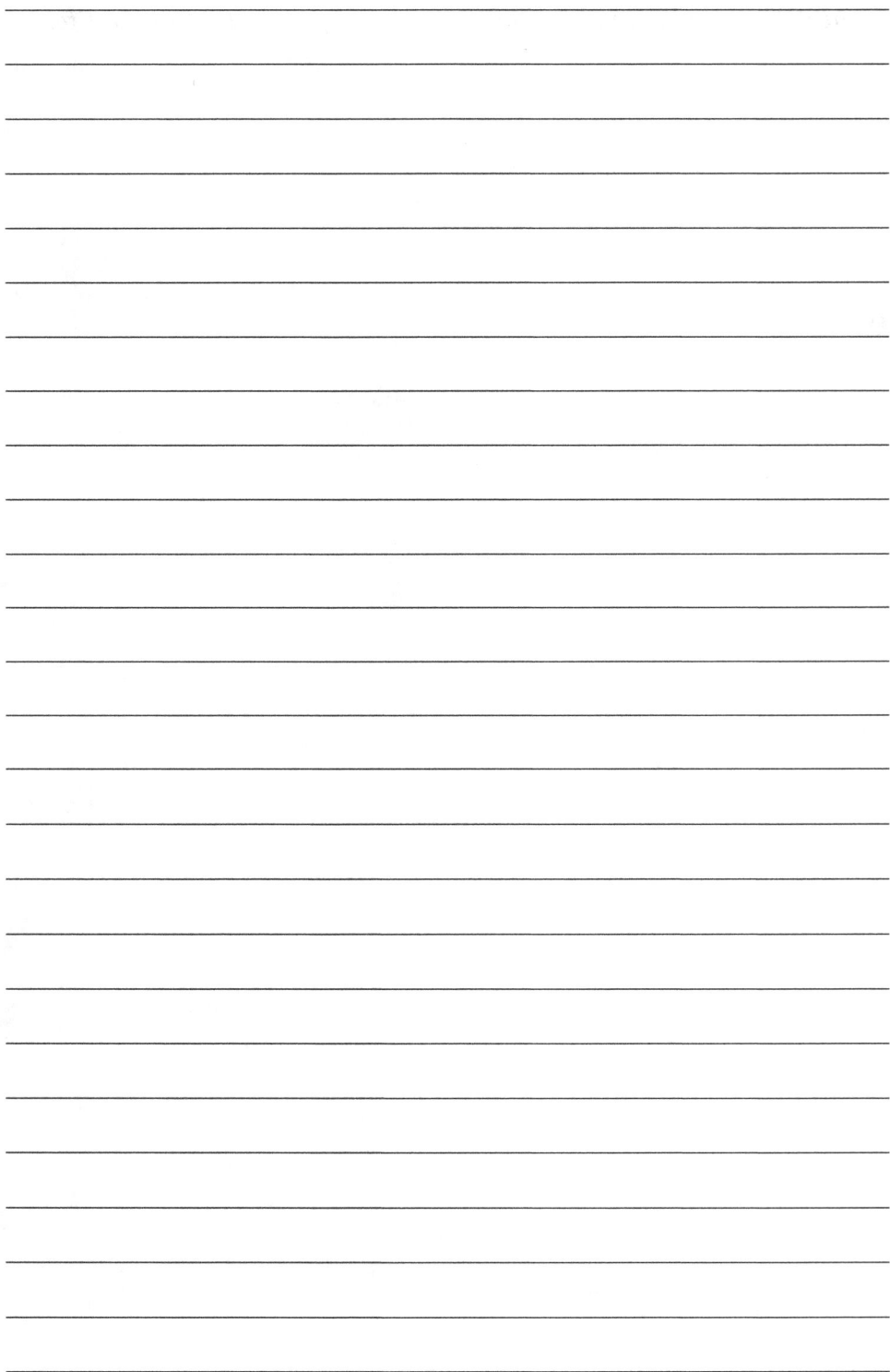

www.ingramcontent.com/pod-product-compliance
Lightning Source LLC
Chambersburg PA
CBHW060456280326
41933CB00014B/2773